The Secret of
The Non Diet
For Children

Rudy Kachmann, M.D.

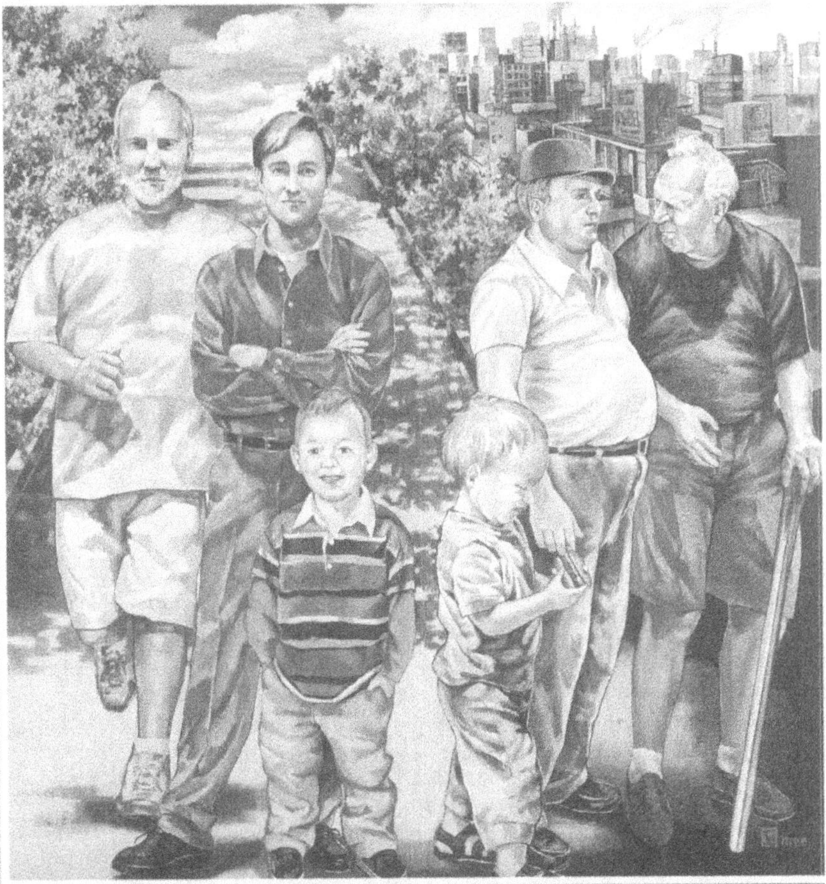

EDUCATE YOURSELF · TEACH YOUR CHILDREN

Published by Rudy Kachmann, M.D. Kachmann Media, LLC
www.KachmannMindBody.com

Library of Congress Control Number: 2009940711

ISBN-13: 978-1503369863 ISBN-10: 1503369862

Cover Illustration by Mee Kyang
Shim Cover design by Kenneth Loechner
Copy Editor, Courtney L. Hartman

Printed in the United States of America

CONTENTS

THE STATE OF OUR CHILDREN'S HEALTH

As many as 35% of American adults are obese and 60% are overweight. The American Heart Association defines obesity as simply having too much body fat as measured by your body mass index (BMI). Your BMI is determined by a formula that assesses your weight relative to your height. An adult who has a BMI between 25 and 29.9 would be considered overweight, while an adult with a BMI between 30 and 39.9, (around 30 pounds or more overweight), would be considered obese. A person with a BMI over 40 would be considered morbidly obese. For example, a man who is 5'9" and weighs between 125 and 168 pounds would have a BMI between 18.5 and 24.9 and would be considered to be at a healthy weight. However, weighing in at 169 to 202 pounds would put that same man in the overweight category with a BMI of 25 to 29.9. He would be considered obese if his weight fluctuated just a few pounds and his BMI was 30 or higher.

Unfortunately, 35% of the population is equal to about 72 million American adults who are obese. That's a staggering number when you consider it's approximately 1/3 of our entire population. Out of that number of people, seven million are morbidly obese. Since 1998, the rate of obesity in the United States has increased almost 25%, and the rate of morbid obesity has grown even faster. In other words, we're fat, getting fatter,

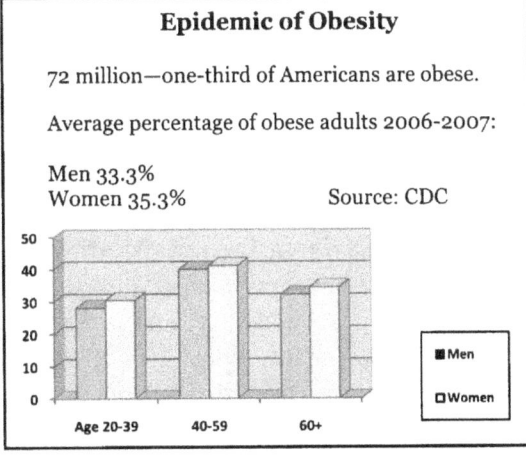

Epidemic of Obesity

72 million—one-third of Americans are obese.

Average percentage of obese adults 2006-2007:

Men 33.3%
Women 35.3%   Source: CDC

Common Inflammatory Diseases
- Alzheimer's
- Asthma
- Cancer (mouth, esophageal, lung, breast, liver, stomach, pancreatic, colon, rectum, ovarian, endometrial, prostate)
- Chronic Obstructive Pulmonary Disease (COPD)
- Coronary Artery Disease
- Crohn's Disease
- Grave's Disease
- Lupus
- Microvascular Disease
- Multiple Sclerosis
- Obesity (see Chapter 6)
- Ulcerative Colitis
- Pelvic Inflammatory Disease
- Psoriasis
- Rheumatoid Arthritis
- Type 2 diabetes

and getting fatter faster. There is no end in sight to our "growth," and there is no indicator that our country will suddenly slim down and get into shape. What's most disturbing is that we're also getting sicker. Obesity is a major risk factor for a host of deadly diseases, including vascular disease, heart attacks, strokes, high blood pressure, certain cancers, inflammatory diseases and other serious health problems. There is a huge group of type 2 diabetics, and the numbers are growing.

Not only are we getting fatter faster, we're getting fatter at a younger age. Since 1990, we have seen a 300% increase in the rate of overweight and obese children in our country. Today, with as many as 32% of American children overweight, childhood obesity is now the most common pediatric disease. Data from two National Center for Health Statistics surveys, 1976 to 1980 and 2003 to 2004, show the prevalence of overweight children ages 2 to 5 years, increased from 5% to 13.9%. For those 6 to 11 years, prevalence increased from 6.5% to 18.8%. And for those ages 12 to 19 years, prevalence of obesity increased from 5% to 17.4%. These numbers represent our nation's youth and future leaders. As a country, we want leaders who will be healthy and able to lead.

To develop leaders, our children need to grow and mature with a healthy self-esteem. Most overweight children will have poor self-esteem, so it is probably true that the most immediate and widespread adverse effects are psychological. However, the long-term effects are clearly cardiovascular and metabolic. Studies from the National Center for Health Statistics also show that obese children tend to grow into obese adults. Once, a study found that 80% of children who are overweight at age 10 to 15 were obese adults at age 25. Another study found that if a child is overweight before age eight, obesity in adulthood is likely to be more severe. In the last year, over one million people have died from vascular disease, including strokes and heart attacks. I predict that number will be 1.5 million within 10 years. We will be in store for serious and expensive medical problems, and many of our children will die young if we don't make some changes.

Unfortunately, too many health care providers tend to underestimate the impact of pediatric obesity, or lack the skills, knowledge and time to treat it effectively. I believe all schools should be required to calculate the BMI and waist measurement of every child. It is also my opinion that employers should be required to check the BMIs of their employees. This is a national standard of practice in Japan due to a huge increase in obesity and the ensuing diseases and healthcare costs. It's not surprising that our healthcare industry is booming while insurance companies, as well as uninsured individuals, struggle to keep up with the rising costs.

Autopsies that were performed on the Korean and Vietnamese soldiers during the Korean and Vietnam wars revealed no vascular disease, with the exception of American soldiers, where the incidence was about 70%. This finding is a true reflection of the ravages of the mad, sad, and often toxic, American diet.

Obesity is a serious problem. But it's a problem you can overcome through diet and exercise. Studies show that approximately 30% of weight loss is directly related to exercise, a well-known fact that I will continue to mention throughout this book.

My goal in writing this book is to educate you on food choices and how to nourish yourself and your children in a way that will reflect a well-balanced and healthy future for your family. This book is not about portion control or calorie restriction. A healthy lifestyle does not have to include starvation or deprivation. "You are what you eat," is a fitting phrase. You literally create your health, or lack of, by what you choose to put in your mouth. By reading this book, you will realize that the old phrase, "fat mamas make fat babies," is also true, not only because of nutrition choices, but because our genes also play a part in our health. Many choose to blame genes rather than change their lifestyles, i.e. regular exercise and healthy nutrition. If your calorie intake is high and you choose high carbohydrate and high fat foods while leading a sedentary lifestyle, chances are you are obese, not because of genes, but choices.

Reportedly, communities of Hispanic and African descent have a gene based on evolutionary history that can be stimulated by bad food, which results in high rates of hypertension, heart disease and diabetes. These ethnic groups need to be especially careful about what they eat and what they feed their children. When I was at Georgetown University and worked at D.C. General Hospital, I treated a lot of African-American patients for brain hemorrhages and hypertension. The cases I saw were essentially all diet related. Unfortunately, the genes they inherit can remain dormant, but they tend to be manifested by the American diet. This theory was proven by a study that was performed in 1956 in Africa. Researchers had a hard time finding a single patient who had reportedly suffered a heart attack. At the time, researchers concluded the African population's diet was more of a vegetarian diet, and this healthy way of eating had positively affected the health of the nation. As a lifetime member of the NAACP, I think the fact that the organization has not made this a priority is disappointing. A healthy lifestyle should be adopted in childhood and should be taught to all new parents, especially minority groups with tendencies toward obesity.

Throughout this book, I will describe a plan for healthy eating without counting calories or portion control. I've had many patients whose diabetes disappeared by following the secrets of the non-diet. By adopting healthy eating habits you will look great, feel great and live a long life!

CHAPTER ONE
SYNDROME X
A SILENT AND DEADLY EPIDEMIC

In the United States, we are in the midst of a disease epidemic bigger than anything we've ever seen. Worse yet, this life-threatening disorder, a malady that experts call a silent killer, is largely unrecognized. An alarming percentage of us, including adults and children, have the disorder and don't know it. It's called Syndrome X and it's the cause of diabetes, vascular disease, cancer and inflammatory diseases.

Syndrome X goes by a number of different names. It is known as Reaven's Syndrome (after Dr. Gerald Reaven, the Stanford University doctor who discovered it), insulin resistance syndrome, glucose intolerance, pre-diabetic syndrome, or metabolic syndrome. The Japanese, who don't like the term obesity, call it "metabo."

Whatever you call it, the disorder refers to the body's inability to properly metabolize the foods that too many of us eat these days - the American diet of fast food, trans fats, high cholesterol meats, cheeses and refined sugars.

Many adults and children have Syndrome X and never realize it, not even when it affects their health in ways that oftentimes go undiagnosed. In fact, as many as half of all adults and one-third of all children have Syndrome X, and most blame their health issues on something else.

What are the indicators of Syndrome X? There are four major symptoms:

1. Glucose intolerance and insulin resistance
2. Obesity
3. Blood fat abnormalities
4. Hypertension

However, you don't have to have all four conditions for a diagnosis of Syndrome X. You only need two. And with 50% of Americans overweight, 50 million suffering from hypertension, and 50 million living with high cholesterol, you begin to see the problem.

Does your child have Syndrome X? Do you? Syndrome X is a nutritional disease, so what you eat and what you feed your child will determine whether or not you have it. If you want to know if you are a candidate for Syndrome X, ask yourself these questions.

- Do you and your children frequently eat chips, doughnuts or pretzels?
- Do you chose to eat hamburgers, hot dogs, fatty lunch meats, fast foods and french fries instead of complex carbohydrates and whole grain foods like potatoes, corn, sweet potatoes, brown bread, vegetables and fruits?
- Do you have close relatives who have diabetes, heart disease and obesity?
- Does your child exercise regularly?
- Would others consider your child a "couch potato?"

By answering the previous questions, you can get some idea of the risk of your child developing Syndrome X. To take it a step further, find out your child's body mass index or BMI. What is your child's waist measurement? Measuring your child's waist and comparing it to the radius of your child's chest and hips can be an accurate gauge in determining the true situation. If your child has a potbelly or if your child's waist is greater in inches than his/her chest or hips, you've got a problem. You can find BMI tables for children in this book on pages 79 and 80.

You will also need to know the level of your child's triglycerides. A healthy level of triglycerides is 150 or lower. In Syndrome X, high levels of triglycerides are caused primarily by a diet high in fat and refined carbohydrates, because they've been stripped of their phytochemicals, fiber, vitamins and minerals. All the healthy elements of these carbohydrates have been removed. In other words, the intake of refined carbohydrate foods will increase your level of triglycerides. The fat your child eats turns into triglycerides, which creates fat cells. An excessive amount of fat cells can lead to coronary artery disease and many other health problems, including Syndrome X. Foods like muffins, doughnuts, white pasta, white bread, cookies, soft drinks, and fatty foods would fall into the refined carbohydrate category. Sadly, this is a large portion of the American diet and our diets are only getting worse!

Worsening Food Habits

Years ago, the average American consumed several pounds of refined sugar in a year's time. Today, the average American consumes more than 150 pounds of refined sugar annually. Simply put, our bodies are not designed to metabolize that much sugar. The amount of sugar we're consuming daily is what leads to Syndrome X, vascular disease, diabetes, cancer and inflammatory diseases. Americans would be healthier and have fewer risks of fatal diseases if they simply changed the way they eat.

Although some diseases are genetic, many can be controlled through healthy diet and exercise. A proper diet, along with daily exercise, cuts down the amount of fat in your body. Fat, especially the visceral kind deep in the abdomen, generates bioactive substances that promote insulin resistance and inflammation affecting every cell in the body especially the sensitive endothelial cells that line the walls of arteries. Specifically, visceral fat cells produce inflammatory cytokines, which trigger inflammation and the production of high levels of CRP. Silent, long-term inflammation can cause even more damage to the artery's endothelium than plaque. Simply stated, fat kills.

Throughout history, a healthy amount of fat in the body has been necessary to help create body heat and to keep the body going during long

Weight-related Conditions
- Acid-reflux, heartburn
- Asthma, respiratory problems
- Back pain, disc herniation
- Cancer: endometrial, breast, ovarian, prostate, colon
- Coronary artery and microvascular disease, angina, stroke, heart attack, sudden death, heart failure
- Depression, eating disorders
- Erectile dysfunction
- Gallbladder disease, gallstones
- Gout
- Dyslipdemia
- Hypertension
- Insomnia, sleep apnea
- Insulin resistance, metabolic syndrome, and Type 2 diabetes
- Osteoarthritis

periods of famine. Today, fat is literally taking over America. As stated earlier, one of the leading causes of fat is refined carbohydrates. Here in the U.S., instead of eating more of the beneficial complex carbohydrates, that are found in fruits, vegetables, nuts and legumes, we are swimming in a sea of highly refined carbohydrates. Our consumption of refined carbohydrates, like processed white bread and bakery products, has increased almost 30%.

Our supermarkets are full of foods that are not grown, but instead are designed and manufactured. New foods are being invented every day, but these invented foods are not good for us. They are so unnatural that if you put many of them in a bag and wait about five years, you'll find that they don't rot.

The bottom line is that the food industry is geared toward highly processed foods that, by their very nature, promote insulin resistance.

Glucose Intolerance/Insulin Resistance

Glucose intolerance and insulin resistance are the main culprits of Syndrome X. Glucose, or sugar, is your body's energy food. Think of glucose as the gasoline that runs your body's engine. Glucose provides energy for everyday activities and for building new body tissue. Every cell in the body requires a relatively steady supply of glucose to function normally. If we don't have enough sugar we become shaky and unsteady. The ideal blood sugar ranges between 80 to 100 mg. Humans have complex biological safeguards that protect us in order to avoid dangerous extremes of low or high sugar levels.

The hormone insulin is necessary for most of the body cells to properly use glucose. Produced by the pancreas, insulin drives glucose into our cells where it is either burned for energy or stored as fat.

Insulin resistance is caused by elevated insulin production and inefficient glucose metabolism. Manufactured, refined foods are high in sugar and raise the insulin levels, resulting in inefficient glucose metabolism.

CHAPTER TWO

THE BOGALUSA HEART STUDY

In 1973 in his hometown of Bogalusa, Louisiana, Dr. Gerald Borenson, a professor of cardiology at the Louisiana State University Medical School, founded a study to investigate the effects of diet and exercise on children. By 1994, in its 21st year, more than 14,000 children had been followed in this study. The oldest child in the program is now approximately 35 years old.

The American Medical Association Journal, as well as hundreds of other medical articles on cardiology, reported on the results in 1992. The study reveals that elevated cholesterol and LDL levels could be found in children as young as six months of age, and those with high levels usually maintain them. There are many markers of vascular disease, elevated cholesterol, high LDL, low HDL, inflammation, obesity, diabetes, lack of exercise, etc. But the mother of all markers is still the cholesterol level, indicating it is as important as the rest of the markers combined. For example, in the famous Framington Heart Study, there were no heart attacks seen in patients who had a cholesterol level under 150. So, you can see that cholesterol is a master marker.

If any children died suddenly of accidents or other similar causes of unexpected death during this study, autopsies were conducted. Fatty deposits, or "fatty streaks," were found in the aorta, the main vessel leading from the heart, on many children over the age of three and in the coronary arteries of most of the 190 children and young adults that were autopsied. Many of these children and adults had been followed in the study for years. Those with the highest known cholesterol levels had the largest amount of fatty deposits, which simply points out the need to control cholesterol levels during childhood. Pediatricians still do not get a cholesterol level of all children. Although this testing is not currently recommended by the American Pediatric Association, I guarantee in the near future it will be - though it may be a bit too late for us by the time they make it mandatory.

A number of other studies have pointed that out that as early as 1930, early signs of vascular disease were found in 30 children in Europe.

These findings, although reported in major medical journals in Europe and America, have been generally ignored by the medical community, and almost completely ignored by the public. Practicing pediatricians and family physicians either pay no attention or are not made aware of the information. I gave a book on pediatric obesity to one of the pediatricians in my medical center and asked him to review it and give me his opinion. One year has gone by and he has not reported back to me. I suspect he's not very interested.

At Johns Hopkins University, they studied a thousand medical students. Those with the highest cholesterol levels at age 20 were three times as likely to have heart attacks and nine times as likely to die of them. Clearly, they followed those medical students for a long period of time. The Bogalusa Heart Study found moderate and high risk cholesterol levels in 40% of 20-year-old to 26-year-old men.

Children at the Highest Risk

Family history plays a part in about 10% of the cases. If family members are dying in their 30s, 40s, and 50s of heart disease, you have to wonder if their cholesterol levels were high at a very young age, and possibly on a genetic basis. Of course, their children should be checked at a very young age, which is recommended by the APA. I recommend checking the cholesterol levels of all children, since the family history of many children is not known. I have seen patients die in their late teens or early 20s from vascular disease, proving that checking levels and cholesterol at a young age is important to long life and health awareness.

In 1991, the Mayo Clinic section of pediatric cardiology found that reducing the saturated fat in the diets of 32 children reduced their average cholesterol levels in only three months, just like in adults. Larger groups of children in an uncontrolled environment, such as schools, have shown similar reductions in their cholesterol levels after both educational and dietary interventions.

Most industrialized nations are experiencing high mortality rates from heart disease. This was not the case just decades ago. During communist rule in China, two doctors from Oxford, Dr. Colin Campbell from Cornell University and a number of Chinese physicians studied one billion people. They found many different eating patterns in different parts of China. The areas that were largely vegetarian had very little vascular disease, very low cancer and low diabetes rates. The China study was extensive and large.

They have traced the Japanese from Japan to Hawaii and into California. They gradually increased the vascular disease rate and cancer rates. The Japanese in California had the same rate of fat disease and cancer as the average U.S. population. The rate of heart disease in the rural villages of China was 26 per 100,000. The rate in the United States was 4,000 per 100,000 - 155 times higher.

African-Americans and Diet-related Disease

The above statement very clearly proves that what we eat is directly linked to vascular disease, diabetes, cancer and inflammatory diseases. Clearly, prevention starts at a very young age. If you want your child to have the best chance in life and have a healthy and long life, you must teach him/her to eat the right food at a very young age. If you eat the same diet, you will also save the rest of your family. If you are the primary shopper, preparer and server of the food in your home, you must set a standard for health in what you eat, in order to be an example to everyone else in your household.

CHAPTER THREE

THE PSYCHOLOGY OF FOOD FOR CHILDREN

To change the way you think about food and, in turn, improve your child's overall health, it's important to realize that food is a drug. When food is digested, it is broken down into several different chemicals. These chemicals have great effects on your brain and body. Some foods increase or decrease your appetite, some affect how you think and feel, whether happy, depressed or anxious. These chemicals include sugar, endorphins, beta-endorphins, serotonin, gaba and so on. For most of us sugar is an anti-depressant, at least for a while. It tones us down, numbs us, slows us and masks pain. Take away sugar and we are anxious, irritable, angry and restless, and have trouble sleeping. We feel less able to cope without sugar. In its own way, it's as good as a drink. After all, alcohol is liquefied sugar.

For some of us food is a lifeline, an essential tool in our emotional survival kit. It takes away stress, numbs our fears and worries and stops the world. It's a womb, a haven, a cave, an escape and a refuge. Eating is an automatic response to feelings that is quickly applied without thought. To break this pattern it takes tremendous sustained effort. Diminishing the power of the bond with food takes a revolution. If food has become a cornerstone to all of your psychology, if you're using it to change your thinking, an equally strong foundation must replace it. If you're using food to reduce stress or improve your mood, you can see the problem. Actually, most of us do that in some way, and some do so in an excessive way. Physical dependence or an addiction to a substance means the body has been altered in a way that makes absence of the substance painful. You can be addicted or habituated to food, just like alcohol and narcotics. There are receptor sites on the cells in the brain that are changed by the chemicals in your food, just like receptor sites are changed by alcohol or drugs. The nerve cells have developed extra receptor sites to adjust to the changing concentration over neural transmitters, like serotonin or endorphins. Neurotransmitters, such as serotonin, jump the gap between nerves and make them work. When food is withdrawn, there are less neurotransmitters and you feel pain, anxiety, irritability and stress. These extra sites may never go away. If you resume eating too much sugar or too much refined food, you often experience weight gain.

Physical addiction to food chemicals occurs when neural functioning and structure are altered as a result of the presence of the chemical. The addictive substance, sugar, has caused an alteration in the organic structure of the body. During this cycle, taking the substance relieves discomfort of withdrawal. This is a strong indicator of physical dependence.

I was sitting in a plane the other day and watched as a 300 pound man, who sat across the aisle with his wife, tore open a huge bag of potato chips with his teeth because he could not open it with his hands. He gulped down the entire contents of the large bag within about five minutes. Thirty minutes later he ate another large bag of chips as he simultaneously snacked on a bag of cookies. Just like a drug addict or alcoholic, he was trying to change the chemistry of his brain with serotonin, endorphins and dopamine. It was very sad to witness, knowing why he had chosen that food to eat and why he couldn't eat enough of it.

From the time we are born, our brains are trained with food chemicals. We cry and we get food. The things that we need for survival, through evolution, have joy and pleasure associated with them. For example, food makes us feel good. Additionally, sex and exercise result in the release of endorphins and give us pleasure. We reward our children with ice cream and cake on birthdays, and we serve deserts at parties and family gatherings.

Being overweight or obese is much more common in stressed families. Families with financial problems, marital problems and those who are lower on the economic scale have a lot more overweight and obese children, and their parents are often overweight. A lot of that has to do with psychology and the chemical effects of the food. And frankly, bad food, high-fat food, processed food, refined food and fast food restaurants are much easier to afford. If your family is on a budget or doesn't have much to spend on food, chances are your diet will not be one that's healthy.

So, changing what you eat and feed your child can affect this psychology. Don't use sugar, processed foods, refined carbohydrates, doughnuts or pretzels to calm them down or regulate their behavior, as they will likely become overweight and obese. Good food habits must be taught at a very young age or they become more difficult to change. Reduce or eliminate sugars, or your kids may become sugar addicts, which many of us are. Remember, sugar releases chemicals in the body, just like alcohol or cocaine.

Is your Child Addicted to Sugar and Refined Food?

Take a few minutes to evaluate your family's eating habits. Using a piece of paper and pencil, write down a few observations. When your child comes home from school, ask what he or she ate for lunch. Take interest in what the school is feeding your child. Are they giving your child a diet high in sugar and refined foods, and just a few vegetables or fruits? Do your kids snack on doughnuts and cookies when they come home?

Take a good look at your child. What is his or her BMI? Look at the charts on pages 79 and 80. Is your child overweight or obese? Only you can change things by educating your children to make the right nutritional choices and by buying the right food. The example you provide to your children will carry over to what they eat when out of your sight. What are your kids eating before they go to bed? Will they eat an apple or banana, or do they normally choose to eat cookies and ice cream? Do the children have a lot of stress? Are they smoking? Smoking is stressful to a young, growing body. Are they using alcohol or drugs?

Most people who are addicted to sugar are also addicted to refined, low nutrient carbohydrates. Refined carbohydrates have been stripped of their coverings that were once full of nutrients and fiber, and they generally appear white in color. White bread and white rice are pure sugar, while brown bread and brown rice still have nutrients and fiber. Fiber prevents absorption of a lot of bad chemicals, and acts as a natural filter for your body. An example of a complex carbohydrate is a baked potato with its skin. It is a very healthy complex carbohydrate, high nutrient and high fiber food.

Serotonin, a chemical in your brain, helps determine how you feel. If your serotonin level is functioning poorly and your life becomes stressful, you get some relief from that stress by eating sugar. Children with a lot of stress do that, as do adults. Once the sugar high stops, you eat again. You may develop a dependency on food through such a process.

When do you stop eating? If serotonin reaches certain concentrations, it's supposed to tell you to stop eating. Some people have a malfunction in this feedback loop and they eat the whole loaf of bread, the whole bag of potato chips, the large tub of popcorn with butter or the whole box of doughnuts, and they can't help it.

Endorphins also make us feel good. Certain endorphins, such as beta-endorphins, stimulate eating. People susceptible to beta-endorphins need enormous quantities of food. A symptom of this problem is difficulty knowing when to stop eating once they've started. Serotonin is known to alter mood, decrease appetite and pain and facilitate sleep.

The hypothalamus, located at the base of the brain, regulates appetite. The hypothalamus contains the functions that have to do with long-term survival, eating, sleeping, aggression, drinking and sex. Survival is pleasure. The basic rule of thumb is: if an activity is important for the survival of the species, it is pleasurable. If an activity is harmful to the survival of the species, it's painful.

CHAPTER FOUR

THE PSYCHOLOGY OF OBESITY

An overweight person is very likely someone who has been using food to tamper with brain chemistry. The tampering occurs because something is wrong with the person's brain, and chemicals that come from food intake are a fast-acting method of altering brain function to temporarily fix the problem. What's wrong with the brain? Recent experimental studies indicate that a malfunction in serotonin functioning may be an important factor in obesity. Serotonin is that neurotransmitter that leads to relaxation and sleep. It's also a stress reducer, anxiety reliever and quick fix for common maladies. Serotonin affects mood and decreases the experience of pain. Some people with low serotonin levels are depressed. Depression has been found to occur in children as well as adults. Without realizing it, children can temporarily alter their brain functions and feel better with the consumption of certain foods. These types of foods are often referred to as "comfort foods."

Oftentimes, parents will see their child sad or depressed about a situation or occurrence and their first reaction is to take the child out for ice cream, bake cookies, prepare their favorite snack or meal or offer them candy. Unknowingly, this instantaneous reaction teaches your child that food will make it all better. Parents don't consider the long-term psychological changes they're instigating in the way their children will react to stress in the future. The child grows up in a cycle of dealing with stress and the pressures of everyday life with food, which in turn, leads to obesity. This cycle of coping is passed down from generation to generation. The cycle doesn't end because the connection is never made between coping, food and obesity without understanding the emotional response and the changes that occur in the brain when coping is done in this manner.

How Sugar Changes Your Brain

It's a well-known fact that carbohydrate intake boosts serotonin release. But most people don't understand that people who crave carbohydrates may eat too many of them in an effort to improve their mood or to correct inadequate chemical levels.

One of the chemicals our brain constantly craves is serotonin. Besides altering brain function, serotonin also decreases the amount of food a person eats. A feedback loop tells the person to stop eating. For some reason, certain people's feedback loop is malfunctioning. These people can eat a loaf of bread and nothing tells them to stop. If you have a disorder in your serotonin function you will experience metabolically caused cravings. Having these types of cravings doesn't mean you're morally weak or undisciplined. Your body is constantly telling you to eat. There is nothing inside your brain that is telling you when to stop eating. You continue to consume the carbohydrates until you can hold no more, often taking in far more calories than you can possibly burn off in a day.

Whatever the reason, chemically caused eating is not your fault. It's a physical abnormality like diabetes and eating the proper food can cure both. The problem is chemically based, so the good news is that you can do something about it. You are not helpless, and neither is your child. As with any disorder or disability, it's important to instill in your child that this is not an excuse to be overweight. There is a solution as long as you are willing to work at it. Not following the little voice in your head that screams to eat ice cream, cake or anything sweet is difficult, at first. But like any lifestyle change, it can be accomplished once the voice of reason takes over and tells you why you're having those cravings. As time passes, it becomes easier to control the urge to eat unhealthy foods.

Science of Cravings

Serotonin is made from tryptophan that's located in the brain and the bowel. Recent studies have shown that most of the serotonin is made in the bowel. When we eat a diet rich in complex carbohydrates the sugar triggers insulin release, which pushes amino acids into the muscles. With that, many tiny tryptophan molecules are now in higher levels in the blood, and they get pushed into the brain and bowel to make serotonin. The serotonin makes you feel better.

If you are over eater, the following is likely:

- Your serotonin level is insufficient.
- This insufficiency may cause you to feel depressed and to be sensitive to pain.
- You crave carbohydrates to correct the imbalance.
- Eating carbohydrates and sweets increases the increased beta-endorphin levels in the blood, which increases appetite.
- Insulin causes muscle storage of amino acids that compete with tryptophan to be carried into the brain.
- Blood levels of tryptophan increase in proportion to competing amino acids.
- Tryptophan enters the brain and bowel.
- Serotonin is manufactured and released.
- You feel better, you feel sleepy and your pain is dulled.
- Nothing tells you to stop eating.

Endorphins

Next, endorphins and enkephalins come into play. They are like morphine, giving pain relief and a feeling of pleasure. As mentioned earlier, these feelings of pleasure and reduction of pain can also lead to cravings. Beta-endorphins are well known for stimulating food cravings. One such endorphin is Dynorphin. Dynorphin is your body's natural defense mechanism. It has many purposes such as fighting the effects of drugs in your system. With the release of a stimulant into your brain, dynorphins are released to lower the pain. A sudden release of dynorphins can be misread as a craving, when it's actually working to alleviate a sudden chemical change, such as in a stressful situation.

The danger of endorphins is they feel good, and we unconsciously find ways to cause their release. One of the easiest ways to release endorphins is with the consumption of sugar. Increased beta-endorphin levels in the part of the brain where it is regulated, the hypothalamus, have shown increased sugar, starch and fat intake. If you overeat, you're chemically stimulated to continue overeating. You're not a wimp. You're not stupid. You have an imbalance of chemicals.

Children that are overweight or obese usually have a history of stress problems originating in the family. Some have picked up bad habits and associate eating with comfort, while some have been abused, which is not unusual in the history of many patients who are overweight. Again, feelings of unworthiness while coping with overcoming abuse can lead children and adults to turn to food as a source of consolation.

A person is probably more vulnerable to the effects of brain chemicals if they been fasting, dieting, or under stress. The body may become physically dependant on these physiologically released chemicals. We may become addicted to our own brain chemicals to trigger the release because they make us feel better. It's like using alcohol or cocaine.

The act of chewing is thought to release another chemical called dopamine. Dopamine is a chemical that is released by cocaine. Cocaine addiction is about dopamine chemical imbalance—the more you chew, the more dopamine is released. This leads to a cycle of constantly finding something to snack on, and with the addition of sugar as your snack, you're releasing more than one chemical into your brain and heightening your eating experience.

Coping with Stress through Food

Many studies demonstrate that mild to moderate stress increases eating, while severe stress usually decreases eating. If a tiger is running at you, your appetite will turn off. But once he is gone and you get worried, the appetite returns. After eating something sweet, like a doughnut, you feel better because the sweet releases endorphins. Acute stress, like being chased by a tiger, or any impending catastrophe, is over quickly. Chronic stress lasts longer and causes us to eat.

We experience stress, and we need a sugar fix. The overeater becomes compelled and driven to get it, like a cocaine addiction, because the relief after eating is so immediate.

People prone to a food addiction may experience pain more clearly and have lower moods than other people because of abnormal chemical functioning. Endorphins and serotonin relieve pain, reduce anxiety and make you feel good, all while you're getting fat. Have you ever heard the expression "Fat and happy"? You now understand the meaning behind that expression.

When you were Born

Even as a newborn, when you were irritable, fussy and crying, your parents gave you food to fix the problem. As you grew older your parents may have used food to deal with their own emotional problems. Human beings learn how to relieve pain very quickly. Food is something that immediately works to stop pain. We were fed and then we cried again. If crying brought mom with warmth and reassurance, we cried again. We ate more sugar, and the more we ate, the better we felt. We did not know we were changing the endorphin receptors in our brains just by crying and eating sugar. But as we grew older we may have noticed that we could eat more sugar than our friends. They would be satisfied with one piece of candy, but we weren't satisfied unless we ate the whole bag. Gradually we became dependant on sugar. Some of us preferred fatty foods and most of us ate sweets, starches and fats.

As the years passed, the addiction became more entrenched. Food became such a focus in our lives that it was more important than anything else. We began to center our lives on eating. We began to plan for what we would do in relation to eating. Every plan, every vacation, every step in our daily lives also took into account what we would have for meals and snacks along the way. We were gaining weight, but not paying attention. We thought obesity was beautiful, but did not realize it was killing us.

Sadly, vascular disease can start as young as age four! Fifty percent of our nation's teenagers have an elevated, abnormal cholesterol level. Many doctors don't check the cholesterol level of teenagers. If your child is overweight, there is a family history of vascular disease, or relatives are dying at young ages from heart attacks and diabetes, have you and your child's blood fat profile checked. Having knowledge of this information is very important!

Basic Emotional Release

All this eating continued to manipulate our brain chemistry as we repeatedly trigger the release of endorphins and serotonin. We did it to relieve pain, and we became addicted to the feeling it gave us. When these chemicals were released, we felt pleasure. Many over eaters have a similar story. Oftentimes they will have a history of low self-esteem and, in more serious cases there has been abuse. A child has many basic emotional needs. If they are not met, many of them overeat.

The following is the science of basic emotional release:

- Oxygen, nourishing and well-balanced meals, fluids, exercise, fresh air, sleep and rest
- Cuddling, holding, loving and respectful, physical touch
- Safety - protection from physical, emotional and sexual danger
- Communication - sharing of thoughts and ideas
- Honesty - words consistent with actions
- Tradition - structure, repetition, security and predictability
- Validation - a sense of a relationship, healthier ways to handle feelings

If a child does not receive the above, they may use chemicals like food, alcohol or drugs to tranquilize their brains. When a child isn't held enough, he or she experiences a deficit. It's horrible if the child is ridiculed, ignored or never asks to be held. It's ghastly if the child asks to be held and is sexually abused. Protection, trust, safety and honesty are needed, whether they are supplied or not. Emotional needs don't go away, but we learn to shut them down or to substitute something else for the true need. Food acts as a substitute for emotional needs. The more children experience shame for having emotional needs, the more they eat. The more they eat, the fatter they get. The fatter they get, the less likely their emotional needs will ever be fulfilled. It's a vicious cycle that starts in early childhood when a child is not properly loved.

The Inevitable Failure of Diets

Diets are systems of food deprivation. It's no wonder the body recoils when it's thrown into the shock of a diet. Food was supplying the nurturing, comfortable state, and it gave a reward that nothing else had. Long-term physical restriction of food will not work because you are not meeting the emotional needs of the person. Sooner or later, the need for comfort and relief will overpower, and even wipe out, all the memory of the motives for dieting. Within a very short time, the food addict will be back on the merry-go-round. Even a little bit of sugar will trigger your obsession with food and sweets.

Alcohol, drugs, sugar and overeating are all effective ways to avoid living and feeling. Once we've learned avoidance, we can automatically use it again. The next stress can trigger avoidance without us ever spotting it. Before we realize what's happening, we're overeating to get the chemicals that make us feel better. We have learned to substitute a substance, food, for real need, affection, love and so on.

Changing your eating habits may take a lot of support from your family. We all have emotional needs and those needs have to be met or overeating will continue. Keep in mind that your job as a parent is to ensure you meet the emotional needs of your child. Parents love, support, protect, raise and teach their children. You should teach your child when to eat by not raising an emotional eater, and by teaching them the correct food to eat.

CHAPTER FIVE

FOOD CHOICES FOR SUPERIOR HEALTH

Your child's health is an issue that needs to be addressed before he or she is even born. In recent years, mothers-to-be have become better educated about nutrition, lifestyle and how an unborn child's health could mirror the mother's. For example, while I was teaching a class at Indiana University-Purdue University on mind-body medicine, there was a student who was at least six months pregnant. She was overweight and had gestational diabetes. Her diabetes started during pregnancy from being overweight. Babies from diabetic and overweight mothers are more likely to be obese and have diabetes, along with other medical problems.

One day, I gave a lecture about proper diet. The student followed my recommendations and lost about 20 pounds. Her diabetes went away and she looked and felt a lot better. She will save her child from a lot of trouble if she continues eating properly. This is just one example of how a mother's health prior to conception can ultimately affect both her health during pregnancy and her child's health. Therefore, it is important to eat healthy prior to conception, as well as after one's pregnancy has begun. Good health habits are extremely important during pregnancy and improve the chances of good overall health for both mother and baby.

Feeding Your Infant

Breast-feeding your baby for the first two years is one of the best gifts you can give your child. Only about 25% of mothers do it, and most stop at six or eight months. Only 16% of infants in the United States are breast-fed until one year of age. This is unfortunate, considering the benefits that breast-feeding offers in regards to health. Giving your child the benefits from breast milk is important, if not critical, in the first six months of life. But don't stop after six months!

Great Grains
- Wheat
- Oatmeal
- Corn
- Popcorn
- Brown rice
- Whole rye
- Barley
- Bulgur
- Millet
- Buckwheat
- Quinoa
- Sorghum

Breast-feeding is recommended to at least 18 months, and preferably up to two years of age.

Infants benefit from breast milk more than packaged formula because human milk contains living cells, hormones, active enzymes, immunoglobulins and compounds with unique structures that cannot be duplicated. By breast-feeding, the spaces between the cells that allow the mother's immunoglobulins to be absorbed gradually get tighter, reducing the potential for food allergies. No infant formula can duplicate human milk because formula does not contain the living cells that are found in breast milk. Despite the list of benefits given by formula manufacturers, human milk is the food best designed for babies. The benefits of breast-feeding far outweigh benefits from any formula on the market.

If parents are seeking to maximize intellectual and health potential, they must breast-feed. One of the main benefits of breast-feeding is that breast milk boosts immunity in children. Your child is going to have fewer infections if he or she receives the immune cells from mother's milk. Babies who are breast-fed are also at a lesser risk for breathing related diseases. Since the mother feeds the baby directly without involving containers, etc. the risk of infection or contamination is practically eliminated.

Did you know that prolonged breast-feeding also reduces the risk of breast cancer? By breast-feeding, both you and your child will see long-term health benefits. Breast milk is high in Omega-3's and other essential fatty acids.

If you cannot breast-feed your child until at least the age of two, a DHA supplemented cow or soymilk formula should be used.

What about Cow's Milk?

Exposure to dairy proteins from cow's milk has shown long-term negative consequences when used early in life. Cow's milk increases the chance of developing childhood diabetes and promotes early life growth spurts linked to later life cancers. Your child does not need cow's milk to be healthy. But, if used at all, it is very important that it not to be started before the age of eighteen months.

Cow's milk, fruit juice and french fries are still commonly given to infants before their first birthday, a major mistake. The first two years of life are filled with opportunities to build a disease-resistant child and to have that child develop healthy eating habits that can last a lifetime. If parents realized how important breast-feeding is for the future health of their child, a much higher percentage would breast-feed longer. We need to teach parents that breast-feeding is important to a child's good health.

The Secret of Enhancing your Child's Brain

The brain is 50 – 60% fat, with mainly omega-3 fat in the cell membranes.

By age of two, the major development of your child's brain cells has occurred. It's the wiring occurs later.

When you are pregnant, and even before you are pregnant, it is critical to follow a healthy diet for maximum brain development of your newborn child. Following the secrets of the non-diet would be a great way to achieve this. Eating omega-3 Thai food months before pregnancy is great.

If you have pregnancy related diabetes or gestational diabetes you must adjust your diet quickly or your child will be seriously affected and will not receive full potential brain development. Be sure to eat plenty of foods that contain omega-3, such as fish and nuts. The fish should be mercury free. I recommend taking supplements of nuts and flaxseed for additional good, essential fatty acids. Sardines have high omega-3's. Pregnant women who eat fish have better-developed babies,

Bountiful Beans

Legumes or beans contain a lot of resistant starch that we digest slowly or not at all. They also have a low glycemic load.

- Adzuki beans
- Black beans
- Black-eyed peas
- Butter beans
- Calico beans
- Cannellini beans
- Edamame
- Fava beans
- Garbanzo beans
- Great Northern beans
- Kidney beans
- Lentils
- Lima beans
- Mung beans
- Navy beans
- Pinto beans
- Soy beans
- Split Peas

less premature births and fewer occurrences of low birth weight babies.

As I stated previously, the best thing you can do for your child is to breast-feed until they are two years old. Breast-feeding will help stimulate the brain in a way that formula cannot. Children who are breast-fed have been proven to be more intelligent since breast milk, not cow's milk, is high in good brain omega 3s and other good fatty acids.

30% of mothers only breast-feed up to six months, which is real loss to the children. A study in New Zealand, found that cognitive ability of the child was often directly related to the length of time the child was breast-fed.

Breast milk can be deficient in essential fatty acids, DHA and omega 3's if the mother eats the wrong food. A typical American mother's breast milk contains much less omega-3 then a typical Asian mother's breast milk because Asians tend to eat a healthier diet. 200mg of DHA as a supplement seemed to bring breast milk to acceptable levels in pregnancy and mothers eating a poor diet.

High-fiber Foods
- Rhubarb
- Spinach
- Sprouts
- Raisins
- Prunes
- Peppers
- Cabbage
- Carrots
- Eggplant
- Kale
- Lettuce
- Corn
- Cauliflower
- Okra
- Onions
- Beets
- Broccoli
- Berries
- Apples
- Cranberries
- Dates
- Figs
- Grapes
- Mangoes

If it is necessary to give your child formula, you can add omega-3 supplements approved by the FDA. No fetal brain, infant brain or child's brain will realize its full brain potential without the essential fatty acid, omega-3.

In the United States, infant formula is not fortified with omega-3's, although some companies are beginning to do it without an FDA mandate. Some states and many physicians, including Dr. Stoll of Harvard University, highly recommend it. Dr. Norman Salem of NIH says there is a consensus that DHA should be added to infant formula to make it more like breast milk.

Studies have proven that infants fed good fats in the first four months of life were more intelligent six months later.

How to do it

- Breast feed your child as long as you possibly can
- Follow the secrets of the non diet before, during and after pregnancy
- Take DHA and omega-3 supplements
- Eat fish at least two to three days a week, eat some sardines, some nuts
- Supplement your infant with DHA. 20mg of DHA for every 2.2 pounds of body weight, 100mg of DHA for a 6-pound baby

Six to Nine Months

In the next six to nine months, introduce new foods gradually. Puree fresh fruits such as apples, pears or peaches. Alternate with vegetables cooked in a pressure cooker or steamed, then pureed. Commercial, organic baby food is a convenient way to serve green peas, carrots, squash, zucchini, string beans and other healthy foods. Grinding up raw nuts and seeds are an excellent source of protein. These also have the healthiest type of fats and are loaded with minerals and vitamins. Many new parents don't think about health foods when their child is ready to eat solid foods. But starting children on these types of food will not only benefit them early in life, but there will also be long-term benefits as children learn to make proper food choices as they grow.

Foods to avoid in the first year are eggs, fish, meat, cow's milk, cheese, butter, oils, fruit juices, honey, peanuts and processed foods with additives or salt.

Trans Fatty Foods
- Biscuits
- Breakfast bars (some)
- Cookies
- Crackers
- Cream
- Doughnuts
- Fried foods (some)
- Pastries
- Lard (shortening)
- Margarine
- Salad Dressing (some)
- Potato Chips

One Year

After the child's first birthday is a good time to begin feeding him or her vegetables and bean soups. Babies under the age of two need adequate fat in their diets. As viable breast milk decreases in quantity after nine to twelve months, add avocados, tofu and nut butters, not cheese or butter, to ensure they get a healthy amount of fat in their diet.

Toddler

After age two, your child can eat healthy table foods like the rest of the family, and supplement healthy snacks, water and juices between meals.

The Picky Eater

I know someone with triplets whose children eat mainly meat products, and they develop a lot of infections. They are picky eaters. They will only eat meat at a restaurant and the parents say they don't need anything else. Children are not responsible for their food choices, but the parents are. Most of the time it's the mother, and occasionally the caregiver, who makes food choices for young children, not the child. A nutritionally poor diet is predominately the result of misinformed parents and incorrect dietary choices. It is not uncommon or abnormal for a child to prefer a narrow range of foods at a young age. It is not unusual for parents to be in an ongoing battle to coax their child to eat in a matter they feel is appropriate. It is possible to put an end to the food wars and solve the problem of getting your child to eat a healthy diet.

Twenty-five percent of children eat fast food french fries daily. Many children who eat the wrong foods are often sick. Many have been on several antibiotics for ear infections and some are always on antibiotics.

Dr. Joel Fuhrman in his book, Disease Proof Your Child, has cured many infections in his patients by teaching mothers the proper diet to feed their children. It is not necessary to coax your

> **Dietary Approaches to Stop Hypertension (DASH):**
> - Emphasize fruits and vegetables. Daily goal is 5 servings of fruit and 4 servings of vegetables daily
> - Choose non or low-fat dairy products
> - Choose whole-grain breads and cereals
> - Eat walnuts and almonds
> - Reduce intake of red meats, sweets and sodas

children to eat healthily. In fact, battling about food with your child is counterproductive. The answer is to only permit healthy food in your home. It even works for me, as an adult. There are no doughnuts or cookies at our home, so I don't eat any. When I come home late at night from a hard day's work, I grab anything I can see. Because junk food is not there, I don't eat it. Your children can do the same. If you only provide healthy snacks, that's what they'll eat.

The earlier in life you introduce good food to your child, the easier it will be to continue a diet of good nutrition and disease prevention as he or she ages. Taste is something you learn. There are no fat receptors on your tongue. You are not born with cravings for fat or junk foods. That is a taste you have to acquire. The message is clear - children raised in an environment of natural foods will more likely continue healthful eating practices as they grow. Scientific investigations illustrate that children most often take on the habits of their parents. If you eat a lot of steaks and fatty foods, so will your children. If you smoke, your child will smoke. If you drink alcohol, your child will drink alcohol.

Adults who consume a lot of fruits and vegetables are usually those who consumed these foods during childhood. My father always ate a lot of fruits, and had fresh fruits available at all times in his deli. I still follow his example at age 72. In short, parents need to eat the same diet they want their children to eat, not only as children, but also into a healthy adulthood.

Don't coerce your children to eat. Let hunger lead the way. Don't concern yourself with the number of calories consumed by your child, unless fatty and high-calorie foods are mostly being eaten. It is especially difficult to get a baby or toddler to eat. Most young children will push food away when they are not hungry. We are designed to consume a diet rich in natural plant fibers and micronutrients. This fiber causes stress receptors in the digestive tract to register that we've consumed enough food. Children will naturally tell you when they've had enough. Concern for pushing away mealtime foods should only be an issue if your child snacks too often, if your child loses weight, or if other health related concerns arise. Otherwise, don't force your child to eat more than he or she needs to feel full.

Old ways of thinking, such as forcing children to clean their plates have contributed to our country's problem with obesity. These work against nature's signals of feeling full and teach children to continue to eat beyond being hungry. If forced to eat everything on his/her plate at a young age, a child will then be programmed to eat what is placed in front of him/her whether he/she is hungry or not, even if he/she has too much food to eat. Large portions at restaurants will be consumed, along with thousands of unneeded calories.

Man-made, high-calorie concoctions have been designed to appeal to children and increase consumption. They do not contain the nutrients needed for good health, and are becoming more predominant in our country. If your child is not given the option to try these types of foods, in later years, they will not have to work to break the junk food habit.

Avoid, and make sure your children avoid butter, juices that are not all natural or contain sugar, potato chips, french fries, doughnuts, sweets, sausages, hot dogs, lunch meats, and smoked and barbecued meats. They are full of trans fats, cholesterol and refined sugar, which lead to disease and obesity.

What Do I Recommend?

I do not recommend dieting. Dieting is food restriction and substitution, and it will not work. Instead, I recommend selecting the correct foods. Usually calorie counting and portion control is then unnecessary because your body is getting proper nutrition from the types of foods that are made to work naturally with your system in proper digestion, absorption and expulsion.

The types of foods you should be eating are:

- Complex carbohydrates
- Whole grains
- Vegetables
- Legumes, all types of beans
- Fresh fruit

If these are the types of foods you and your child eat, you will be at a proper weight and you will avoid a lot of illnesses and diseases, especially cancer, vascular disease (strokes and heart attacks), diabetes and autoimmune diseases. Plus, your family will enjoy many other benefits. On top of the other, life-saving benefits, every member of your family will look great!

CHAPTER SIX

VEGETARIAN, VEGAN, FLEXITARION—
WHAT DO THEY MEAN?

You may be familiar with the term vegetarian, but what about vegan and flexitarion? All three mean something very different. A vegetarian avoids meat and products made from meat while a vegan avoids meat and dairy and foods made from animal byproducts. A flexitarion way of eating is a combination of the above. About 70 to 80% who follow these plans choose a vegetarian or vegan way of eating.

The American Dietetic Association, A.D.A., and the Canadian Dietetic Association, C.D.A., have said that a vegetarian or vegan diet is completely compatible with good health. The benefits include normal weight, little vascular disease, a reduced risk of cancer, reduced infections, reduced autoimmune diseases and a very healthy lifestyle. You and your child will look good and have no psychological effects from being obese.

Summary of the Secrets of the Non-Diet

Secret number one—Complex carbohydrates have a lot of fiber, which are large chains of sugar. These chains make it difficult for the body to break them apart, which is ideal for weight control. If you eat one hundred calories of complex carbohydrates, such as baked or sweet potatoes, vegetables, carrots or broccoli, only about 60% of what you consume is ever utilized in the body. A good 25% never leaves the gastrointestinal tract, because of the fiber. Fiber acts as a filter. Refined sugars, white bread, white rice and food stripped of its fiber and nutrients will be absorbed at a 90% rate and raise your blood sugar quickly. So, all calories are not alike. If you eat 100 calories of fat, 97% will sit in your abdomen or buttocks by the next day, only 3% will be used up while metabolizing. This has been proven by needle biopsies.

Complex carbohydrates satiate hunger and turn on our internal furnace, burning calories as heated energy. High sugar, high fat and simple carbohydrates increase hunger, addiction and cravings.

Risk of Complications
Controlling elevated blood pressure can cut strokes by 35 to 40 percent and heart attacks by 20 to 25 percent (Source: AHA)

Secret number two—The same complex carbohydrates that prevent disease can stop, and even reverse, disease.

Secret number three—The resistant starch and fiber in complex carbohydrates absorb fat and defy digestion, while providing few calories.

Secret number four—Refined carbohydrates reduce good HDL cholesterol and increase bad LDL triglycerides, insulin, blood pressure and fat stores. All are proven culprits in the development of inflammation and vascular disease.

Secret number five—Calories are burned faster when they come from foods such as complex carbohydrates. Bodies lose only 3% of the calories from fats, and 10% of the calories from simple carbohydrates. In contrast, bodies lose 40% of the calories from complex carbohydrates, making them the better choice if you want to burn more calories.

Secret number six—Carbohydrates increase tryptophan, an essential amino acid that helps increase serotonin, which reduces appetite and increases feelings of well-being.

Secret number seven—Eliminate olive oil and other vegetable oils while trying to cut back on calories and lose weight, and then use only sparingly. A teaspoon of ground flax seeds can be added to foods as it has the benefits of omega-3 fatty acids without the fat.

Secret number eight—Consuming 100 calories of fat converts into 97 calories of body fat, only three calories are metabolized and drop off. Fat is also an appetite stimulant. The more fatty foods you eat, the more fatty foods you want.

Secret number nine—Reducing fat, but increasing refined carbohydrates works against your goal to lose weight and prevent, stop or reverse vascular disease.

Secret number ten—It is easier for you to change your diet and lifestyle if you avoid restaurants. Restaurants offer larger portions than you typically eat at home, and tempting menu items tend to be full of fat. You should also avoid consuming alcohol because it is 100% sugar.

Secret number eleven— Saturated fat increases inflammatory chemicals, raising the risk of vascular disease, heart attack and stroke. They also increase cancer and infections in children, especially ear infections.

Secret number twelve— Animal proteins have a significant effect on raising cholesterol levels. Plant proteins lower cholesterol levels.

Secret number thirteen—A balanced vegetarian diet has all the protein you need without the cholesterol found in meat products.

High-Glycemic Foods
- Bagels
- Cake
- Candy bars
- Couscous
- Cranberry juice cocktail
- French fries
- Jelly beans
- Mashed potatoes
- Pancakes
- Refined breakfast cereals
- Strawberry jam
- Sugar-sweetened beverages
- White bread
- White pasta
- White rice

Secret number fourteen—It takes 50 calories a day to maintain a pound of muscle. The more muscle you have, the faster your metabolism will be, and the greater number of calories you will burn at rest.

Secret number fifteen—Choose raw foods such as carrots, cauliflower, green peppers and other vegetables. Eat these vegetables raw to lose weight faster. Snacking on crunchy vegetables slows the speed of digestion, making you full for longer periods of time and provides 20,000 phytochemicals, vitamins and antioxidants.

The point of all these secrets is that all foods are not alike. Dieting, which is food restriction, does not work. If you feed your child the correct food, portion control is not necessary. You don't need to act like the food police if you teach your child what to eat. Buy healthy foods and your child will get hungry and eat what is available to them. Look at the school cafeteria and speak to the school dietitian to make sure they're not feeding your child a sad, toxic, American diet. You must take control if you want a healthy child.

Choose a Healthy Lifestyle over Medication

The lifestyle choice I'm outlining in this book is a very healthy way of eating. Dr. Joel Fuhrman would tell you that your child would have fewer infections by following a healthy lifestyle with good nutritional choices and exercise. Remember that very few physicians utilize lifestyle and dietary modifications to treat and prevent illness. A prescription may be the first thing they hand you. We live in a pill and remedy orientated society. Instead of treating the cause, doctors tend to deal with the symptoms. If your doctor wants to give your child an antibiotic, ask for a culture to see if there is actually an infection.

Overmedicating leads to resistance to medications. When medicine becomes necessary, a stronger medicine with sometimes dangerous side effects must be prescribed to penetrate the resistance that's been built up by taking unnecessary medicines. Oftentimes, medication is unnecessary, but some doctors react with their prescription pad instead of investigating the cause. Ask your doctor to investigate before medicating, especially when it comes to your child.

Healthy Choices

Unfortunately, people are looking for a magic cure, rather than getting the root of the problem. We become what we eat, and our future health is dependent on how carefully we build our bodies with optimal nutrition and minimal exposure to dangerous chemicals and toxins.

Start in your home with a variety of produce, especially fresh fruits, raw vegetables, and raw nuts and seeds. Don't turn your child into a steak eater. He/she may develop a high cholesterol level and an increased risk of vascular disease. Eventually, he/she may also become obese. Replace most foods of animal origin with foods of plant origin. Bean burgers, vegetable and bean soups, and fruit-based desserts are great choices. If you continue to eat meat products, use only white meat such as poultry and eggs a few times weekly, and other animal products less frequently. Use only the white of the egg and throw out the yolk. Limit sweets and remove sugar, salt, white flour and all products with these ingredients from the home. Don't turn your child into a sugar addict! Remember that sugar is in foods that you use daily such as ketchup, white flour, white bread, pasta and some cereals that are portrayed as healthy. Your child can become addicted to sugar without eating sweets by eating these condiments and foods. Instead of eating ketchup, make your own tomato sauce with fresh produce. Instead of white flour, bread or pasta, choose whole grain.

When eating dairy foods, select non-fat varieties such as fat-free milk. In general, it's best to reduce dairy consumption. A cow does not drink its own milk. It's not a necessary part of a healthy diet. Milk is not a health food after age two. As your child grows, milk is not needed for calcium. Only 30% of calcium from milk is absorbed. There is adequate calcium in vegetables.

As a timesaver, use a very large pot to make vegetable soups with beans. That same soup can be eaten for several days after it's made. By not adding animal products, you won't have to worry about food spoiling as fast or the meat turning sour. Cooked soups with vegetables and beans tend to stay edible longer than soups with meat.

In North America, about 70% of our dietary protein comes from animal foods. That's why half a million people die every year from heart disease, and another half a million from strokes. You only need about 30 to 50 grams of protein a day, yet Americans consume about 120 grams of protein a day.

The cholesterol-lowering effects of vegetables and beans are proven. When adult subjects were fed a vegetable-based diet, cholesterol levels dropped radically, much more than with the most powerful cholesterol-lowering drugs.

The foods with the most nutrients per calorie are vegetables and beans. Vegetables are very rich in protein and calcium. Most vegetables have more protein and more calcium per calorie than milk. Green vegetables and grains have more proteins per calorie than meat. One hundred calories of broccoli have twice as much protein as one hundred calories of meat. Vegetables and whole grains have all of the eight essential amino acids, as well as the twelve nonessential amino acids. You don't need to eat meat to get these amino acids. There has been some question about the amount of B12 in vegetables. To satisfy everyone, I recommend taking a B12 supplement.

A proper way of eating will drop your cholesterol as fast as medication over a two to three month period of time. Meat can be very expensive too. Think about the money you would save by eating this way.

CHAPTER SEVEN
CONTINUATION OF THE SECRETS

A nutrarian is a person who has a preference for foods that are high in micronutrients, vitamins and minerals. This is a great way to eat. Some low-fat meat is allowed, chicken without skin, white turkey and some low-fat fishes. Dr. Joel Fuhrman has found that children who eat a nutrarian diet have fewer infections. This is a good alternative if your family is accustomed to eating meat because the change is less drastic. At first, the foods might taste strange, look unappetizing and some members of your family may grumble and groan at mealtime. With consistent efforts, your child will eventually give in if there is nothing else available. They will learn to like healthier foods. Be consistent!

Some people believe they cannot tolerate healthy food, or their children will not tolerate it. Statements like, "They only eat meat," should not be believed. Anyone can change. Dr. Joel Fuhrman called this Inflexible Palette Syndrome. An inflexible palette is one that is believed to not tolerate healthy foods. This assumption prevents people from believing they can change their lives. We, indeed, can change. We eat the wrong foods out of habit. By constantly eating the correct food, old habits die, often within two to three weeks. It's been shown that 21 days of consistent, changed behavior and forcing of new habits will reprogram you into making a change in your life, no matter how engrained the habit is in your daily ritual. You simply have to reprogram the way your whole family eats so you can support each other in making these changes. If the parents continue eating a poor diet, the children will have a hard time changing. It takes a community of loving, educated, informed and motivated people to make a change. Who would want their child to start in last place, die young, have a stroke or heart attack at a young age, be ridiculed by their classmates or develop cancer at a young age? Nobody wants that, so please make the changes that are necessary so your child doesn't fit into one of those categories 10, 20, or 30 years from now.

As I mentioned earlier, you should also speak to the school dietitian. Are they buying the surplus cheese from the government? Cheese is the most saturated fat-dense food there is. A lot of schools buy surplus from the government because it is more affordable. Can you imagine that the government subsidizes these farmers to produce the very food that is killing us? It makes no sense.

You must take control if you want a healthy child with a great future. Do you want your child to be living in a nursing home at age fifty? If you keep feeding him/her the sad, toxic, American diet, it very well may happen.

Fats to Avoid	
Saturated Fats: Butter, cheese, whole milk and ice-cream; meat; snack foods; chocolate bars; coconut and palm oils	Saturated fats raise total blood cholesterol as well as "bad" LDL cholesterol.
Trans Fats: Partially-hydrogenated vegetable oil; French fries; baked goods; margarine	Trans fats raise LDL cholesterol and lower "good" HDL cholesterol.
Fats to Use Sparingly	
Monounsaturated Fats: Olive, peanut, rapeseed, and canola oils; peanut butter; avocados; cashews, walnuts and almonds	Monounsaturated fats lower total cholesterol and LDL cholesterol and increase the HDL cholesterol.
Polyunsaturated Fats: Soybean, safflower, corn, and cottonseed oils; walnuts; fatty fish	Polyunsaturated fats also lower total cholesterol and LDL cholesterol. Omega-3 fatty acids belong to this group and have the unique quality of reversing plaque.

Percentage of Specific Types of Fat in Common Oils and Fats*

Oils	Saturated	Monounsaturated	Polyunsaturated	Trans
Canola	7	58	29	0
Safflower	9	12	74	0
Sunflower	10	20	66	0
Corn	13	24	60	0
Olive	13	72	8	0
Soybean	16	44	37	0
Peanut	17	49	32	0
Palm	50	37	10	0
Coconut	87	6	2	0
Cooking Fats				
Shortening	22	29	29	18
Lard	39	44	11	1
Butter	60	26	5	5
Margarine/Spreads				
70% Soybean Oil, Stick	18	2	29	23
67% Corn & Soybean Oil Spread, Tub	16	27	44	11
48% Soybean Oil Spread, Tub	17	24	49	8
60% Sunflower, Soybean, and Canola Oil Spread, Tub	18	22	54	5

Values expressed as percent of total fat; data are from analyses at Harvard School of Public Health Lipid Laboratory and U.S.D.A. publications.

THE SECRETS OF THE NON-DIET

1. SECRET: All carbohydrates are not alike. Starchy, complex carbohydrates quell hunger and turn up our internal furnace, burning calories as heat and energy. High-sugar, high-fat, simple carbohydrates increase hunger, food addictions and cravings.

2. SECRET: The same starchy carbohydrates that prevent disease and premature death can stop and even reverse disease.

3. SECRET: The "resistant starch" in complex carbohydrates absorbs fat and cholesterol, and defies digestion while providing few calories and the feeling of fullness.

4. SECRET: Refined carbohydrates reduce the "good" HDL cholesterol and increase insulin levels, triglycerides, blood pressure and fat stores—proven culprits in the development of inflammation, obesity, diabetes and vascular disease.

5. SECRET: Foods that promote weight loss are high in complex carbohydrates which take more energy (calories) to break down. Your metabolism speeds up to process the critical nutrients of these foods. A faster metabolism can burn excess body fat.

6. SECRET: Consumption of complex carbohydrates helps the brain produce higher levels of serotonin which reduces your appetite and increases your feeling of well-being.

7. SECRET: Reducing saturated fat without reducing refined carbohydrates works against the goal to lose weight and prevent or reverse chronic disease.

8. SECRET: Saturated fats increase artery-clogging LDL-cholesterol. The unsaturated fats in oily fish, walnuts, flaxseeds and plant-based oils reduce LDL-cholesterol, inflammation and plaque within blood vessels.

9. SECRET: Trans fat offers what the Mayo Clinic calls "the cholesterol double-whammy:" it raises "bad" LDL-cholesterol and lowers "good" HDL-cholesterol. The greater the percentage of trans fat in a food product, the higher risk is for heart attack and stroke.

10. SECRET: Try to eliminate olive and other cooking oils while trying to lose weight, and then use them sparingly. Fish or a teaspoon of ground flaxseeds or walnuts offers the benefits of omega-3 fatty acids without all the fat of oil.

11. SECRET: Animal protein raises cholesterol while plant protein lowers it. Meat also raises artery-clogging saturated fat.

12. SECRET: To get the minimum amount of protein you need each day, balance your vegetables with beans and (if you're not on a diet) nuts.

13. SECRET: To lose weight faster, choose raw foods such as apples, carrots, cauliflower, bell peppers and other whole fruits and vegetables eaten raw. Snacking on crunchy foods slows the rate of digestion and provides thousands of disease-fighting nutrients.

14. SECRET: It takes 30-40 calories a day to maintain a pound of muscle. The more lean body mass you have, the faster your metabolism will be, and the greater number of calories you'll burn at rest.

CHAPTER EIGHT

THE DIETARY RECOMMENDATIONS OF THE AMERICAN PEDIATRIC ASSOCIATION, THE A.P.A., AND THE AMERICAN HEART ASSOCIATION, THE A.H.A.

When we look at the typical diet that Americans have been eating, we have to wonder, where was the government? Where was the American Pediatric Association? Where was the American Medical Association? Where was the Surgeon General of the United States? The White House, even under President Clinton and President Bush, had a new chef every few months. They could have been teaching Americans the proper way of eating. For the whole country to change, the leaders must lead, that means from the president on down. We need a Surgeon General who promotes wellness throughout the entire country.

In August of 2005, the American Pediatric Association and the American Heart Association revised their 1982 recommendation. Would you say it was about time when we are leading the world in vascular disease, adult diabetes and cancer? They also state the atherosclerotic process begins in youth, culminating in the development of vascular plaque in the third and fourth decades of life. Although, you must remember that autopsies done on our young soldiers reveal vascular disease in 18, 19 and 20-year-olds. But in foreign soldiers, the numbers are very different.

The new focus is on both total calorie intake and eating behaviors. Calorie-dense foods and beverages with minimal nutritional content must return to the role as occasional discretionary items in an otherwise balanced diet. The present recommendations are based on strong scientific evidence. I agree with most of it, but not all of it. More on that later.

The following are some of their recommendations.

Table 1

A.H.A. pediatric dietary strategies for individuals aged greater than two. Recommendations for all patients and families:

- Balance dietary calories with physical activity to maintain normal growth
- 60 minutes of moderate to vigorous play or physical activity daily
- Eat vegetables and fruits daily, limit juice intake
- Use vegetable oils and soft margarines low in saturated fat and trans fatty acids instead of butter or most other animal fat in the diet.
- Eat whole grain breads and cereals, rather than refined grain products
- Reduce the intake of sugar sweetened beverages and foods
- Use non-fat-skim or low-fat milk and dairy products daily
- Eat more fish, especially oily fish, broiled or baked
- Reduce salt intake, including salt from processed foods

My Opinion

I agree we should eat more fish, however I think there should be more discussion about how much and what type of fish is best to eat. Dr. Joel Fuhrman would say, "Fish is not a health food." I agree. It's too fatty, and contains a lot of contaminant chemicals, mercury, PCBs, and so on. Eating fish twice a week is plenty. It shouldn't be consumed seven days a week.

Also, at what age do we not need milk, even the low-fat variety? Breast-feed until the age of two, after that it's not needed. Certainly a limited amount of low-fat milk seems reasonable.

Table 2

Tips for parents to implement AHA pediatric dietary guidelines:
- Reduce added sugars, including sugar sweetened drinks and juices
- Use canola, soybean, corn oil, sunflower oil and other unsaturated oils in place of solid fats during food preparation
- Use recommended portion sizes on food labels when preparing and serving food
- Use fresh, frozen and canned vegetables and fruits and serve at every meal. Be careful with added sugars and sauces, read the labels.
- Introduce and rightly serve fish as an entrée
- Remove the skin from poultry before eating
- Use only lean cuts of meat and reduced-fat meat products
- Limit high-calorie sauces such as Alfredo, cream sauces and hollandaise
- Eat whole grain breads and cereals rather than refined products. Read labels and ensure that whole grain is the first ingredient on the food label of these products.
- Eat more legumes, beans and tofu in place of meat for entrées
- Breads, breakfast cereals, and prepared foods, including soups, may be high in salt and/or sugar. Read food labels for content and choose high-fiber, low-salt and low-sugar alternatives.
- More physically active children and adolescents would require additional calories.

My Opinion

Emphasis that's different from the past includes the allowance, and also more liberal intake of unsaturated fat, and a focus on ensuring adequate intake of omega-3 fatty acids. Essential fatty acids are needed to build membranes and brain cells. This is just as I recommend. There's an emphasis on foods that are rich in nutrients, and that provide increased amounts of dietary fiber.

The A.H.A. continues to recommend diets low in saturated and trans fats. Healthy foods include fruits, vegetables, whole grains, legumes, low-fat dairy products, fish, poultry and lean meats. Again, I am concerned that there is no recommendation on the amount of fish that should be consumed.

Also, there seems to be no limit on the use of vegetable oils, they are very fatty, and sometimes are 100% fat. A pound of olive oil or canola oil is heavier than butter. Plant derived oils have a lot of calories.

Removing the skin from poultry is fine, but it doesn't say how many days a week you can eat it. Eating chicken seven days a week is not healthy, with or without the skin. Some people think it is healthy. Chicken is 40% fat. When I look around the doctor's lounge, I get the point. They serve chicken, almost every day. After much prodding, they have finally added vegetarian options.

Table 3

How Many Calories Should a Child Eat?

- One-year-old male and female – 900 calories
- Two to three-year-old male and female -1,000 calories
- Four to eight-year-old female 1,200 calories, male 1,400 calories
- Nine to thirteen-year-old female 1,600 calories, male 1,800 calories
- Fourteen to eighteen-year-old female 1,800 calories, male 2,200 calories

My Opinion

There is a large difference in the amount of calories recommended among sedentary, slightly active and active children. More physically active children need more energy from food to maintain normal growth. But you also have to keep track of their BMI. If you guess and get it wrong, they become overweight. With increasing activity, the discretionary calorie amount may increase by 500 calories a day. If your child is on the football team, he will need more calories than a child who plays video games all day. It all depends on the age and gender of the child, and the level of their activity.

Don't fatten up your child so he can be the center on the football team, he may die at a young age. Your child's health should always be put before your own sense of pride in his accomplishments.

To be active, have a nutritionally adequate diet, and avoid excessive calorie intake in a contemporary society is difficult.

CHAPTER NINE

CONTINUATION OF RECOMMENDATIONS
OF A.P.A. AND A.H.A.

Age Two to Six Years

At this stage, recommendations for diet content are similar to those for older individuals. Your focus should be on providing quality nutrient intake and avoiding excess calories. My personal opinion would be if you watch the nutrients, you don't have to worry much about the calories, except under unusual conditions. Dairy products are a major source of saturated fat and cholesterol in this age group. Therefore, a transition to low-fat milk and other nonfat or skim dairy products is important. I would suggest that you consider cutting out all milk. No primate drinks the milk of another species. Adult cows don't drink their own milk. Regardless of what has been taught in the past, dairy products are not necessary to health, only the economy.

Sweetened beverages and other sugar containing snacks are a major source of calorie intake. Beverages that are packed with calories are known as "empty calories." They provide no nutritional value and can be replaced with water for better nutrition. They are essentially wasted calories and unnecessary, except to fulfill cravings for sugar or a specific taste. If your child doesn't drink water, and instead drinks sodas or juices, eliminate the empty calories to see an immediate difference.

Table 7 provides a list of strategies for managing nutrition in young children. Parents should remember that they are responsible for choosing foods and deciding when and where are eaten. The child is responsible for whether he or she wants to eat and how much. I would not recommend acting on parental impulses to force children to eat and restrict access to specific foods because they often lead to overeating, dislikes and paradoxical interest in forbidden items. We could agree or disagree about that forever.

Healthcare providers must provide useful advice to parents by going to the A.P.A. and A.H.A. They are constrained by time pressures in the typical health-maintenance office visit, and do not take the time to properly educate about good nutrition and healthy lifestyles. I have been a physician for 40 years and I strongly disagree with the information that is being widely practiced by family physicians and in pediatrician's offices. Wellness must be a way of life. Proper eating must be the first words out of every healthcare provider's mouth. That is the only way things are going to change. We must know the BMI of every patient. We must measure their waist and height and track those measurements on a graph, which could easily be done with modern software and computers. Every patient's weight and BMI should be on the front of their chart and should be tracked with each visit. The health benefits would be tremendous.

Table 7

Improving Nutrition in Young Children

- Parents choose mealtimes, not children
- Provide a wide variety of nutrient-dense foods such as fruits and vegetables, instead of high energy, nutrient-poor foods such as salty snacks, ice cream, fried foods, cookies and sweetened beverages
- Pay attention to portion size. Serve portions appropriate for the child's size and age
- Use nonfat or low-fat dairy products as sources of calcium and protein
- Limit snacking during sedentary behavior in response to boredom, and particularly restrict use of sweet beverages, snacks, juice, soda and sports drinks
- Limits sedentary behaviors, with no more than one to two hours per day of video games or television. No television sets in children's bedrooms.
- Allow self-regulation of total caloric intake in the presence of normal BMI
- Have regular family meals to promote social interaction and a role model for food related behavior

My Opinion

I would agree with most of the advice from Table 7. However, I would add that the best source of protein is vegetables, not dairy products or meat. One hundred calories of vegetables have twice as much protein than 100 calories of meat. Also, if your child is eating a nutrient-rich diet, you have to do very little in regards to portion control, especially if your child is of normal weight.

Age Six and Above

As children grow up, sources of food and influences on eating behavior increase. Social constraints on families may necessitate eating out, influences at school, peer groups, and the increase of fast food intake can all affect choice. At this point, you should educate your child to be a bit picky about what he or she eats. Many children, because of parental work schedules, find themselves home alone and they must prepare their own snacks and meals. You have to have the right food available and teach proper nutrition.

By early adolescence, peer pressure begins to trump parental authority, and fad diets may be initiated. Many meals and snacks are routinely obtained outside the home, often without supervision. Sites include schools, friend's homes, childcare centers and social events. Outside my grandchild's middle school, I noticed a huge soda pop machine. Many of the drinks have 50 calories of sugar in them - a quick road to disaster. I have no idea how the school ever allowed it. I suspect it's about money or ignorance, and not children's health. Older children have discretionary funds to use for self-selected foods. This can be very dangerous if they are not educated.

When teens are away from home, their eating patterns do not at all resemble the standard. Unless your child's school has a health-conscious cafeteria, it's best if you can provide at least breakfast, dinner and a single snack at home, where you can monitor what is eaten. It would be ideal if your child could eat every meal at home, but that's rarely possible. You really have to guard your children. Many children do not eat breakfast, and they get at least one third of their daily calories from snacks. The intake of sweetened beverages contributes to total caloric intake. Snacks often contribute to excess consumption of discretionary calories, and supplement the intake of foods containing essential nutrients.

Adolescence is a developmental stage in regards to nutrition, because growth rate accelerates. Amplified caloric needs, due to pubertal growth, stimulate the appetite, but you need to keep track of BMI and be realistic about your child's weight. Being overweight or obese is not beautiful, although there are certain ethnic groups that think so. This is especially sad, because many of them carry a weight-gaining gene, based on evolutionary history, which would never manifest itself unless they eat the wrong food. Look around at the different ethnic groups and you'll get the idea. Realism is important, or you end up with an overweight or obese child. The combination of centrally driven appetite stimulation, and an increasingly sedentary lifestyle due to the decline of regulation sports participation augments obesity. A common example is the transition from high school to college. It is typical for college freshmen to gain about 20% to 30% of their weight via pressure to conform, partly driven by media promoted fast food. These promotions and peer pressure make overeating seem natural.

Currently, increased intake of sweetened beverages, french fries, pizza, fast food and hamburgers has resulted in a subsequent lack of consumption of recommended fruits, vegetables, dairy foods, whole grains, lean meats and fish. This change in eating results in the consumption of excess fat, saturated fat, trans fat and added sugars, along with insufficient consumption of micronutrients such as calcium, iron, zinc, potassium, vitamin C and folic acid.

Keep close track of your children when they transition from high school to college. When they visit home, have them step on the scale and bring them back to reality.

Parental role modeling is important in establishing children's food choices. Current dietary practices in readiness to change must be understood. If you can't get the job done, you may need to hire a dietitian who knows what they're doing and knows how to motivate people.

Schools have become a battleground for fighting the obesity epidemic. I don't know of any school that does this. But, I believe that every school should know the BMI of every child and measure the height and weight of each student at least every six months. This is a public health problem. We pay high taxes for poor health, and the taxpayer should have some rights. Cafeterias are under attack for serving unhealthy food, yet the food provided is constrained by budgetary concerns. Dietary issues are largely external to public health concerns. The US Department of agriculture is not the best at giving good guidelines. They are influenced by politics, especially the farm lobby, the milk industry, the food industry, and heavily by the refined food industry (they spent millions). The proper way of eating is barely mentioned in most schools, especially colleges. Each new college student should know their BMI and their waist measurement, and it should be checked twice a year. The school nurse needs to be educated on proper eating and develop a system of passing information to the students.

Table 8

Strategy for Schools

- Identify a champion within the school to coordinate healthy nutrition programs
- Establish a multidisciplinary team, including student representation, to assess all aspects of the school health Index, or some similar assessment system
- Identify local, regional, and national nutrition programs. Select those that are effective - www.actionforhealthykids.org.
- Develop policies that promote student health and identify nutrition issues within the school - www.nasbe.org/healthyschools/healthy-eating.html
- Work to make healthful foods available at school and school functions by influencing food and beverage contracts that have marketing techniques to influence students to make healthy choices
- Maximize opportunities for all physical activity and fitness programs: competitive and intramural sports, utilize cultures, teachers as role models
- Lobby for regulatory changes that improve the school's ability to serve nutritious food
- Ban food advertising on school campuses

My Opinion

As difficult as it is, the major sports teams should not be the main focus. Sports, where everyone in every class participates, should be the main focus. Physical education programs are often subject to budget constraints. They are actually the most important classes a student can take, if they include teaching proper eating habits. I'm happy to hear that several states have adopted to lead this and are mandating that school staff report to parents the health status of their children.

Table 9

Types of Legislation Under Consideration to Improve Children's Nutrition

- Restriction of certain types of food and beverages available on school grounds. Taxation of specific foods or sedentary forms of entertainment
- Measurement of the BMI by school staff for health surveillance and/or report information to parents
- Establishment of local school wellness policies using a multi-disciplinary team of school staff and community volunteers to educate the parents
- Food labeling regulations, including appropriate descriptions of portion sizes, sugar and fat content of drinks and food

My Opinion

I especially agree we should consider taxing bad food. It might change how we eat. It could also raise a lot of money for schools and healthcare.

Table 10

Consensus Guidelines for Diagnosis of Hypertension and Dyslipidemia and Children

- Pre-hypertension-systolic or diastolic blood pressure > 90th% for age and gender or > than 120/80

CHAPTER TEN

Table 11

Consensus Guidelines for Diagnosis of Hypertension and Dyslipidemia and Children

- Stage one hypertension—systolic or diastolic blood pressure greater than 95th percentile for age and gender on three consecutive visits. Or 140/90mm HG, whichever is less
- Stage two hypertension—systolic or diastolic blood pressure greater than 99th percentile plus five mm HG for age and gender or 160/110 mmHG, whichever is less

> Total cholesterol, mg/dl
> Borderline >170
> Abnormal >200
> LDL-cholesterol, mg/dl
> Borderline >100
> Abnormal >130
> Triglycerides mg/dl
> Abnormal >200

- Increased intake of soluble fiber is recommended as an adjunct to the reduced intake of saturated fat and cholesterol. This is recommended especially for children with a family history of dyslipidemia in an elevated fat profile as a child.

Summary

Essentially, the above was a summary by A.P.A. and A.H.A. of nutrition updates and recommendations for the promotion of cardiovascular health among children and the prevention of multiple other diseases including, and especially, diabetes.

My recommendations of the vegetarian, vegan, nutritarian and flexitarian ways of eating fit easily with these scientific recommendations. My approach is a bit stricter, and probably foretells the future. It is satisfying to see that the A.P.A. and A.H.A. put forth realistic changes since the early 80s, though they are slow to come. The entire nation needs to get involved. The general health of America is not good. We lead the world in diabetes and heart disease, as well as cancer. If these new recommendations were followed, if the present Surgeon General would lead the way and teach the nation how to lead a healthy lifestyle, America would see a better future.

My Opinion

Triglycerides	<	150
Cholesterol	<	150
LDL	<	70
HDL	<	50 for women
	<	40 for men

CHAPTER ELEVEN

NUTRIENT DENSITY—THE MAIN SECRET

The nutrient density of your food predicts your future weight, appearance, longevity and health. Foods contain macronutrients: carbohydrates, protein and fat; and micronutrients: fiber, phytochemicals, minerals and vitamins. So you're getting nutrients and calories from macronutrients, and micronutrients have no calories. All of the calories you ingest come from macronutrients, and micronutrients are very important to your health. The gold standard for weight loss is to eat mainly those foods that have a high proportion of nutrients to calories, as mentioned earlier.

Now that you've learned what those foods are, you have made the first step on the path to good health. The more micronutrients you eat, the healthier you will become. Vegetables, fruits and legumes fit that bill. These foods contain the chemicals that turn the appetite off. You eat less when you eat these nutrient-dense foods at each meal. They will effectively blunt your appetite and you will lose weight permanently. As you consume larger and larger portions of health supporting high-nutrient foods, your appetite for more nutrient-dense foods decreases and you gradually lose your addiction to the unhealthy choices. But you have to commit yourself to doing it right.

The secret is not to eat empty calories. Junk foods are empty calories, their nutrient density is low and they have been stripped of their fiber, phytochemicals, vitamins and minerals. That's why they are called processed foods. In the process of making them last longer, spread further and taste better, everything good and natural is stripped from their base. It's the ingestion of these rich, high calorie foods, while remaining inactive that accounts for weight gain. Remember, exercise is at least 30% of weight loss.

Also, some of us are born with "thrifty genes" based on evolution, African-Americans and South Americans are prone to have these, and

Some Lower Energy-Dense Foods		
Food	% water	Calories/100 g
Navel Orange	85.97	49
Red Grapes	80.54	69
Watermelon	91.45	30
Iceberg Lettuce	95.07	15
Vidalia Onion	91.24	32
Green Pepper (sweet, green)	93.89	20
Watercress	95.11	11
Spinach	91.40	23

Figure 4: Lower energy-dense foods. These foods are high in fiber and water content and low in calories. Lower energy-dense foods are also good sources of vitamins and cancer-fighting ingredients such as antioxidants. (Source: USDA)

eating the wrong foods easily manifests into obesity, especially in children. The Pima Indians in Mexico who eat high nutrient foods are quite thin, have no diabetes and vascular disease. But, the Pima Indians of Arizona have a 90% diabetes rate. The Pima Indians have been studied for over 40 years. Being overweight is not just a cosmetic problem; it leads to vascular disease, a short lifespan, diabetes and cancer. Being overweight is not caused by how much they eat, but what they eat: high nutrient versus low nutrient. Eating large amounts of all the right foods is the key to success and is what makes the secret of the non-diet work. Don't eat anything that walks, runs or flies or you will live in the sky.

Vegetables and fruits are low-calorie foods that have high nutrient density. They contain large amounts of essential vitamins and minerals. They make the calories you consume count toward good nutrition by providing more for the caloric share of the nutrients you need. You should eat at least four servings of fruits and vegetables per day. Beans give you more protein value for your dollar than any other food and are a much better source of protein than meat. Don't eat anything that has a mother or a face. Don't eat anything that crawls, walks, runs or flies in the sky. Being vegetarian has been a part of the human diet for at least 4,000 years. Most of the cultures that choose this type of diet have little cancer and vascular disease.

Starches are not fattening, because fiber will break up about 60% to 70% of starches, and they are metabolized. A number of recent studies indicate that the body wastes more of the calories derived from complex carbohydrates than those that come from protein foods. Complex carbohydrates seem to stoke the body furnace, causing more calories to be burned up as heat. Up to a third of carbohydrate calories that are not digested are excreted, unabsorbed. This is true only of complex carbohydrates. Refined carbohydrates are absorbed up to 90%.

How to Get Children to Eat Vegetables

- Get the children involved in vegetable and salad preparation, as much and as often as possible. They're more likely to eat something they helped make.
- Teach your kids how to cook.
- Teach them how to tear the lettuce apart, and how to cut tomatoes.
- By age four most children can safely handle a paring knife, and can learn to snap beans, slice cucumbers and zucchini.
- Children can grate carrots.
- Take them with you when you shop for food, teach them why you're purchasing healthy foods, and show them how to pick out good produce.
- Use raw, crunchy or steamed vegetables for snacks.
- Prepare healthy, low-fat dip frequently.
- Teach children how to prepare a dip, not ranch but a healthy, low-fat, nondairy choice.
- Come up with interesting ways to serve vegetables.
- Give them funny names.
- Always serve a lot of fruit.
- Frequently make salad the main dish.
- Always ask about what they are eating at school.
- Talk to your children about proper food choices while away from home and explain the difference between healthy eating and junk food.

CHAPTER TWELVE

EXERCISE

Exercise is a very important part of wellness. In adults, it's about 30% of weight loss and maintenance. In children, it's even more important, as much as 30 to 50%. But for an overweight child, exercise can be torture. That's why the topic of exercise must be handled with sensitivity and understanding.

The best way to start an exercise program for your child is to look into the child's unique interests—walking, skiing or tennis perhaps. I remember an overweight child seeking out one of my tennis friends who was the high school tennis coach in Peru, Indiana. The boy said his friends were making fun of him and he wanted to learn the sport. My friend asked, "Are you willing to practice two to three hours a day?" The boy answered, "I will." By the time my friend was finished with him, he made it all the way to the Notre Dame Tennis Team.

Not all overweight children who take up sports will become star athletes. As parents, we shouldn't put those types of expectations on a child who isn't naturally drawn to sports. His/her lack of interest or ability could disappoint, causing a drop in self-esteem. However, you never know what activity might spark interest in your child.

Exercise and Body Fat

Cholesterol levels may be reduced by a low-fat diet, but excess body fat is not necessarily controlled without regular exercise. Active children rarely become overweight.

A regular routine of 60 minutes of cardio exercise will help your child's body burn off the excess fat. Regular aerobic exercise raises the metabolic rate to such a degree that during the remainder of the day and night, more calories are burned per minute, even during rest. You burn calories while you sleep.

Lack of Exercise Equals Neglect

The overweight child, whose parents are waiting for him/her to slim down as he or she grows older, is actually a victim of neglect. By not encouraging your child to participate in sports or physical playtime activities from a young age, you are neglecting your child. You're not encouraging your child to grow into a healthy, secure adult.

A sedentary lifestyle must be addressed as early as possible. It's imperative at a young age that your child is encouraged and taught to enjoy physical activities. Make exercise fun! If you hate exercise, so will your child. If you want a healthy, secure child, you must find a physical activity that you can enjoy together by either participating with your child or taking your child to the activity and cheering him or her on.

There are many activities you can try, but exercise, walking, cycling and swimming are best. And a minimum of three times per week is ideal to get the maximum results.

Once your child is exercising, the attention should be turned to the reduction of total body fat with a high nutrient diet. Avoid empty calories, refined foods stripped of their phytochemicals.

Physical Activity Guidelines

- Provide opportunities for safe, active play inside and outside the home
- Expose children to as many different kinds of physical activity as possible
- Enroll children in sports clubs
- Organize physical activities with the entire family at least once a week
- Encourage walking or cycling to and from school
- Encourage walking the stairs rather than taking the elevator
- Involve the children in home activities such as cleaning their rooms, doing the dishes, gardening or walking the dog
- Limit time watching television or playing computer games to less than two hours per day
- Only allow children to watch television if they have been physically active for at least one hour that day
- Don't allow televisions and computer games in children's bedrooms

School-based Programs

- Provide classroom health education related to healthy nutrition and physical activity
- Involve parents through meetings and educational materials sent to the home
- Provide physical education classes that total at least two hours per week
- Provide active opportunities for break times before, during and after school
- Provide a variety of sports and lifestyle activities
- Promote active transport to and from school, such as walking and bike riding
- Prepare healthy school lunches, low in fat and rich in fresh vegetables and fruits
- Teach the avoidance of sugar filled drinks
- Provide teacher training on the key physical activities, eating concepts and behavior changes
- Provide overweight children the opportunity to participate in a clinic-based weight management program with the cooperation of the parents

The goal of all weight loss programs should be the reduction of body fat. Education of proper diet and exercise in schools can help to make that change.

Schools as Settings for Promotion of Physical Activity

Children spend six hours a day for nearly 40 weeks of the year at school. Thus, it seems logical to utilize the setting for the promotion of healthy, physical activity at schools. They have the necessary infrastructure to do so.

Primary school children should accumulate a minimum of 60 minutes, and up to several hours, of age-appropriate physical activity on all or most days. Children become less active as they mature, so assuring that youngsters receive 60 minutes a day accounts for a likely decrease in activity levels as they age.

Each day children should be involved in 10 to 15 minutes of moderate to vigorous activity. This activity should alternate with brief periods of rest and recovery. Research shows that physical activity mirrors the release of growth hormones and that one's environment exerts a strong influence on physical activity. Sedentary parents produce sedentary children, active parents have active children.

Energy Expenditure - How to Measure it

We can measure the amount of energy used in any activity by using the metabolic equivalent or the "met." The energy of one met is about the same as the energy that is used by the body when it is just sitting still or at rest. The greater the number of mets, the greater the amount of energy used up. The more energy used for the activity, the more calories your child will use up doing it.

One met is one calorie per minute. Walking takes three mets, jogging uses six mets. The greater the number of mets, the harder it is to do the activity.

> Walking = 3.5 mets
> Bicycling = 4 mets
> Dance – jazz or ballet = 4.8 mets
> Skateboarding = 5 mets
> Snow shoveling = 6 mets
> Mowing the lawn with a push mower = 5.5 mets
> Playing the drums = 4 mets
> Basketball = 6 mets

Weight training is another good physical activity. Resting muscle uses up 40 calories a day, at rest. So, having more muscle burns a lot of calories every day. Resting fat only burns three calories a day - a big difference!

CHAPTER THIRTEEN
SELF-ESTEEM

Eating is an automatic response to feelings. What is an overweight or obese child to do when classmates ridicule him/her or make snide remarks? When children are overweight, the opposite sex rejects them. What do they do? Oftentimes, they eat!

When living such a life of rejection and ridicule, anyone, adult or child, will turn to food. They start eating because it's the acceptable drug of choice. Serotonin, dopamine, and endorphins are feel-good drugs produced by the metabolizing of food. A quick trip to a fast food restaurant is a cheap and easy fix for stress because stress is relieved by sugar. This causes the person to feel better while destroying their health and creating a pattern of craving unhealthy food. When sugar is eaten excessively, over time, the nerve cells alter in a way similar to cocaine addiction. Without knowledge of this process, if sugar stops the pain, he or she will soon eat again.

Most children who overeat have serious, profound deficits that have led to painful losses and years of suffering. This leads to low self-esteem.

Low Self-Esteem and Abuse

The lower a child's self-esteem is, the more serious the abuse he or she has suffered, according to psychologists. Child abuse can happen in the child's home with a trusted adult or at school or on the playground with other children. Taking a stick to a child is abusive. Screaming at a child that he or she is stupid for asking that a need be met is abusive. Many children have been beaten and some sexually abused, and overeating is a common response to abuse. To a child, distance, coldness, abandonment and non-interaction are abusive. Poor parenting results in a fearful child, and often manifests itself into fear of abandonment. If you want your child to have healthy self-esteem, you must ensure that he or she has every need met and fulfilled.

Basic Emotional Needs of Children

- Trust
- Affection
- Safety
- Boundaries
- Communication
- Honesty
- Attention
- Tradition
- Validation
- Individuality

A parent who is overwhelmed with their child's needs, depressed or addicted to drugs or food will have difficulty helping his or her child. Food addicts are addicted to sugar. They suffer from mental deprivation. A child watches the parent and if the parent turns to food for solace, then food rescues the child as well.

An addiction to food causes extra weight. Extra weight reduces self-esteem. We think it demonstrates lack of moral strength and that everyone else thinks that since we eat we are weak. "I eat too much." "I smoke." "I take drugs." We think, "Others think that I have no control because I am mentally and morally weak." Again, this causes a loss of self-esteem.

We eat too much to feel better and the excess weight causes us to feel worse. Our children repeat the same cycle. We fear abuse of our children because of their weight, the taunts and the rude, intrusive comments from ignorant loved ones or strangers, those overlooking their own problems, changing the focus from their own mistakes to our children's deficits. We fear discrimination from the club, the group, sports teams and supposed friends. Our children attend school dances with no dates. They grow up with a fear of rejection. No one finds them attractive. They can't find a place to sit because of fear, "Do I fit into this seat or booth?"

Excessive weight fosters isolation and rage. Our kids stay home and get no exercise. They spend their free time playing on computers and video games, or texting. They hide because of lack of self-esteem and their self-image is destroyed. Many people of a large size feel small inside. They hide behind the fat like it's a curtain. It drives people to radical weight-loss products and diet schemes instead of sensible changes and the Non Diet solution.

Do you want your child to live that kind of life? You're here to protect your child and foster a healthy self-esteem, but what will happen twenty or thirty years down the road when your child is in the big world of judgmental, uncaring strangers? Do you really think his or her sense of humor and loving spirit will make a difference to passing, ignorant people?

Anger, compulsions, depression, withdrawal and overeating are the answers for many. Don't let them be the answer for your child. Meet both their emotional and physical needs and foster a healthy, active lifestyle.

CHAPTER FOURTEEN

WHAT CAN THE GOVERNMENT DO?

Look around at the restaurant, the movies and the airport. Watch what people are eating and then look at their body size and shape. What people order for meals, typically matches their size. Some people choose to eat bacon, gravy, egg or doughnuts for breakfast! You can see the results just by looking.

America is in trouble! Two-thirds of our adults and 50% of our children are seriously overweight. Americans are now officially supersized, overweight, obese and, as the Japanese would say, "metabos" (for metabolic syndrome).

Yes, they are generally labeled as being chunky, husky or plus-sized by the clothes manufacturers who are putting larger and larger sizes on the children's racks. Some children are too overweight for their car seats. They're uncomfortable when they squeeze into their little desks at elementary school. Childhood obesity has become a national medical crisis.

As already mentioned, over the last thirty years obesity rates have doubled among preschoolers and tripled for those ages six to eleven. Children are paying a terrible price for this. Diabetes has become a childhood disease. Pediatricians are seeing high cholesterol, high blood pressure and other grown-up problems in children.

Sleep apnea used to be an adult disease where the fat in a person's neck chokes them while they're sleeping, resulting in early deaths, hypertension and heart disease at a young age. I see it in my practice all the time. The answer is not a contraption that you wear at night. The answer is weight reduction.

What Can Our Communities and Governments Do?

The fast food and junk food industries have worked hard to get into the schools. Get them out! Junk food companies have been remarkably strategic about plotting an assault on the schools. The companies have promised underfunded school systems a share of the tag from vending machines, all outright cash gifts. Many school systems have caved in. They're teaching children to die young.

According to a 2005 report by the Government accountability office, 83% of elementary schools, 97% of middle schools and 99% of high schools sell junk food from vending machines or school stores. Parent groups and other critically minded people are beginning to fight back, trying to remove junk food from schools. There are too many states allowing the industry to sell sweets, sugar and bad food at the schools, which is adding to the growing adolescent waistline.

First, Congress should pass a law prohibiting the sale of any foods that are too high in fat, sodium and sugar. The biggest benefit would be to stop the sale of drinks and snacks from vending machines, or any other outlet in our nation's schools during school hours. The U.S. Department of Agriculture should be able to regulate all food being served in schools. State and local school districts should also uphold high standards. A child who has chosen to eat a sugary snack during lunch, or drink a soda is less attentive and oftentimes sleepy afterward. If schools want their students to excel, they'll pay more attention to the children's nutritional needs. Children are a captive audience for the food industry. They will go with the norm, good or bad. If it's not available to them, peer pressure won't cause them to eat or drink foods that wouldn't be available to them at home.

Second, upgrade the school snacks. We need to eliminate the unhealthy snacks and substitute healthy choices. Fruits and vegetables should be readily available in schools.

Third, we need to educate the parents and the teachers about healthy eating. California has been a pioneer, launching a rigorous anti-obesity program in schools. In For the past three years, Arkansas has been weighing children in schools and sending home confidential notes to parents whose children are overweight. We need a national program and I think President Obama is up to the task. Like in Japan, every employer should calculate the BMI and measure the waist of every employee. Every school should be required to monitor the BMI of every child. Then, finally, we may begin to get a handle on the obesity problem. We cannot afford to have a nation where 50% of the people are diabetic; the cost is going to be astronomical.

Fourth, we should start subsidizing healthy food for poor people. Another key reason children are eating badly is that junk food is cheap. We need to tax junk food and subsidize healthy food. If you tell a low-income family, "You really ought to eat more salad and fresh produce," it will essentially encourage them to spend more money on healthier foods. Through the food stamp program, we should give more benefits for buying healthy food, and penalize the recipient for eating unhealthy food. After all, we're probably paying their medical care through Medicaid, and we should have the right to say something about where they are spending our tax dollars.

Fifth, stop subsidizing junk food. We subsidize farmers to the tune of $40 billion dollars a year for growing corn, which is used to make high-fructose corn syrup, a very unhealthy trans fat that leads to vascular disease and diabetes. This subsidy should be stopped immediately, and the money applied to healthy food.

We Need a Fat Tax - I Like to Call it a Fairness Tax or Health Surcharge

America has a long tradition of "sin taxes," cigarettes and alcohol, for example. Why not apply a sin tax to all bad food, fat, sugar, salt, trans fats, beef, high-fat cheeses and so on. The tax would not have to be very high, and we would probably raise billions of dollars, with which we could pay for the health insurance of the nation. If you don't want to pay the tax, eat better food. Though, I would recommend that instead of calling it a tax, we should call it a health surcharge. With a people-friendly title, it may be more widely accepted by the public and congress.

With the additional funds, I think we could pay for Medicare for everyone. The employer would no longer have to buy health insurance for employees. It would make us much more competitive in the world, and we would have a healthier nation. Let's call it a fairness tax or health surcharge. I think people would accept it because they would have insurance and not be worried about the cost of healthcare. Just as federal gas taxes are earmarked for highway construction, fat taxes could be earmarked for special programs, like insurance and so on. The health surcharge would apply to our health insurance.

The junk food companies would fight back hard, but I think we have a president who is willing to step up to the plate. There is no need for us to pay out farm support for bad food, but we should give tax support to good food.

Chapter Fifteen
How did we get to the Western diet?

How is it that America leads the world in vascular disease, strokes and heart attacks, cancer, hypertension, diabetes type II, metabolic syndrome, and adult and children's obesity? It is the American diet.

The health implications for the 21st century are tremendous, including the cost. Horrible illnesses, early death and disability are a huge financial burden that the country cannot afford.

The evolution of the Western diet started about 10,000 years ago. It began when we started farming and domesticating animals. We used to have difficulty hunting and catching animals because we had no guns. And those animals had very little fat on their bodies. Now, we confine them in a pen or cage and feed them to fatten them up before we eat them. That's why we're gaining weight, and why our cholesterol levels are high. Plant food has no cholesterol. Then we started farming, and stripping the good nutrients from the food through processing. This type of processing food was widely popularized approximately 150 years ago. The process turned highly nutritious food into empty calories— foods without vitamins, minerals and phytochemicals. We then started consuming a lot more these processed foods, and we started getting bigger.

When we stopped chasing and foraging for our food, we became more sedentary and less active.

These changes have occurred in too short of an evolutionary time span. Our physiology and metabolism have not been able to evolve and change. Our systems cannot deal with the amount of different foods we are eating. Our bodies have not had enough time to adjust to the foods presented to our physiology. The result is an increase in Western diseases. Those people who have followed a vegetarian, vegan, flexitarian or nutritarion diet have fewer Western illnesses. These diseases of civilization have emerged because of discord between our ancient, genetically determined biology, and nutritional, cultural, activity patterns of contemporary Western populations.

The new way of eating that has developed in the last 10,000 years is characterized by:

- Increase in the glycemic load, much more sugar in the food
- Americans are eating a diet consisting of 30 to 40% fat - it used to be about 10%
- Micronutrient density is much less: vitamins, minerals and phytochemicals have been stripped from the food through processing
- The macronutrient density has changed: much more fat, much more protein and more refined carbohydrates
- Increased consumption of fat had put a lot of strain on the liver and kidneys; acid-base balance has changed because of more protein
- Sodium-potassium ratio is much higher. We are consuming a lot more salt
- Fiber content of food is reduced. Fiber filters a lot of the bad chemicals, such as cholesterol and fats

Evolutionary Discordance

Evolution, acting through natural selection, represents an ongoing interaction between our genes and the environment over the course of many generations. Because only 10,000 years have passed, great evolutionary changes have not occurred and we are getting sicker every day. The diabetic population will double within 15 years if we don't change how we consume food.

In the United States, chronic illness and health problems are partially, if not wholly, the result of what we are eating, probably about 90% of the time.

Chronic disease incidence

- 64 million Americans have cardiovascular disease: strokes and heart disease
- 50 million Americans are hypertensive: high blood pressure
- 30 million Americans have type II diabetes, and the numbers are increasing
- 37 million Americans maintain high-risk total cholesterol concentrations of more than 240
- 40 million Americans have metabolic syndrome that leads to diabetes, vascular disease and cancer, many of those affected are children
- 40 million Americans have osteopenia: low calcium, leading to osteoporosis and broken bones

Now that we understand what poor eating habits can do, we can begin lead healthier and happier lives. Once we understand the value of a healthy and long life, we can develop a purpose and goal and begin to take action.

CHAPTER SIXTEEN
IS MY CHILD OVERWEIGHT?

The subject of overweight and obesity are especially sensitive issues, when speaking of children. Fat, chubby and obesity are not pretty words, and we should not use them, if possible. Whenever possible we should say "overweight" or normal or healthy weight. Healthcare professionals in the US have decided that children in the 90th percentile have a healthy weight and normal level of body fat. Those in the next 5% (the 95th percentile) are considered overweight and those in the last 5% (the 100th percentile) should be considered obese. A healthy weight can be defined as having a body fat level within the normal range that is associated with healthy growth and well-being. Overweight means having a certain amount of excessive body fat is associated with present or future health problems.

An accepted procedure for measuring levels in the child's body is the body mass index, which I'll describe in detail and teach you a way of using at home. Measuring the waist at the umbilicus is the next best method.

The body is made of four main types of material that are responsible for creating your weight - water, protein, minerals and fats. The largest component of body weight is water, comprising about 70% of the body's weight.

How to measure the BMI

You need a measuring tape, weight scale, and the body mass index tables provided in this book. They are different for boys and girls in different for ages.

Instructions

1. Stand up straight with your back against the wall, remove your shoes and socks and look straight ahead.
2. The parents record the date, age, height, and weight in kilograms, or pounds, or centimeters, or inches.
3. Make measurements about every three weeks, recorded in a small book, keep the BMI chart in the book

BMI charts were originally made by calculating the BMI for a large group of healthy children and plotting the measurements on separate graphs for boys and girls, according to age. The BMI charts that give your child's body fat percentiles tell you how many, in the group of children the same age as your child, have higher or lower body fat. For example, if your child's BMI is at the 95th percentile, then their body fat is higher than 95/100 children who are the same age and sex as your child

You can measure BMI with a mathematical calculation, using your calculator.

BMI = weight divided by height squared-height/weight squared, in centimeters or inches, in kilograms or pounds.

Steps for measuring BMI percentile

1. Find your child's age along the scale at the bottom of the chart
2. Move straight up until you find the level of the BMI scale that is the same as what you measured
3. Notice of percentiles are written to the right of the chart, for example 50, 75th, 90th, etc.
4. Recorded percentile onto the weight, height, and BMI chart

Interpreting the BMI percentile

1. Between the 85th and 95th percentile your child is at risk for being overweight
2. Above the 95th percentile would be considered living overweight and some would say obese. The greater amount of excess body fat, the greater the chance the child will have health problems.

In a few cases when a child is very active, with large muscles and large bones, a high BMI may be due to muscle weight or bone weight and not excessive body fat. This is not common, but must be considered.

For adults, a BMI between 18 and 24 is considered healthy, a BMI of 25 to 29 is considered overweight and 30 or higher is considered obese. A BMI greater than 40 is considered morbidly obese. The most common location for women to put on excess fat is around the hips and thighs, giving the woman a pear-shape. Men tend to take on an apple shape, which is more dangerous because fat is around the internal organs.

Measuring the waist has some value, but there are no good reference tables available yet. An individual is commonly measured at the nipple line, umbilicus or the hip line. The measurement of the hips or nipple line should be larger than at the umbilical area.

Growth and development during childhood years is generally characterized as slow and gradual, however marked changes in physical size, shape and body composition occur during puberty. During adolescence, both genders have significant body weight increases with the weight velocity of girls occurring approximately six to nine months later than the height velocity. In boys, changes in height and weight occur at the same time.

I would make sure that during every doctor visit, a nurse measures height and weight and that the doctor evaluates your child's BMI. Teaching prevention and wellness is part a pediatrician's job.

Body Mass Index Table for Children

Form Should be used with accompanying BMI charts from CDC.

Height (inches)	| Normal 19	20	21	22	23	24	| Overweight 25	26	27	28	29	| Obese 30	31	32	33	34	35	36	37	38	39	| Extreme Obesity 40	41	42	43	44	45	46	47	48	49	50
											Body Weight in Pounds																					
25	17	18	19	20	20	21	22	23	24	25	26	27	28	28	29	30	31	32	33	34	35	36	36	37	38	39	40	41	42	43	44	44
26	18	19	20	21	22	23	24	25	26	27	28	29	30	31	32	33	34	35	36	37	38	38	39	40	41	42	43	44	45	46	47	48
27	20	21	22	23	24	25	26	27	28	29	30	31	32	33	34	35	36	37	38	39	40	41	43	44	45	46	47	48	49	50	51	52
28	21	22	23	25	26	27	28	29	30	31	32	33	35	36	37	38	39	40	41	42	43	45	46	47	48	49	50	51	52	54	55	56
29	23	24	25	26	28	29	30	31	32	33	35	36	37	38	39	41	42	43	44	46	47	48	49	50	51	53	54	55	56	57	59	60
30	24	26	27	28	29	31	32	33	35	36	37	38	40	41	42	44	45	46	47	49	50	51	52	54	55	56	58	59	60	61	63	64
31	26	27	29	30	31	33	34	36	37	38	40	41	42	44	45	46	48	49	51	52	53	55	56	57	59	60	62	63	64	66	67	68
32	28	29	31	32	34	35	36	38	39	41	42	44	45	47	48	50	51	52	54	55	57	58	60	61	63	64	66	67	68	70	71	73
33	29	31	33	34	36	37	39	40	42	43	45	46	48	50	51	53	54	56	57	59	60	62	64	65	67	68	70	71	73	74	76	77
34	31	33	35	36	38	38	41	43	44	46	48	49	51	53	54	56	58	59	61	62	64	66	67	69	71	72	74	76	77	79	81	82
35	33	35	37	38	40	42	44	45	47	49	51	52	54	56	58	59	61	63	64	66	68	70	71	73	75	77	78	80	82	84	85	87
36	35	37	39	41	42	44	46	48	50	52	53	55	57	59	61	63	65	66	68	70	72	74	76	77	79	81	83	85	87	88	90	92
37	37	39	41	43	45	47	49	51	53	55	56	58	60	62	64	66	68	70	72	74	76	78	80	82	84	86	88	90	92	93	95	97
38	38	41	43	45	47	49	51	53	55	57	58	62	64	66	68	70	72	74	76	78	80	82	84	86	88	90	92	94	97	99	101	103
39	41	43	45	48	50	52	54	56	58	61	63	65	67	69	71	74	76	78	80	82	84	87	89	91	93	95	97	100	102	104	106	108
40	43	46	48	50	52	55	57	59	61	64	66	68	71	73	75	77	80	82	84	86	89	91	93	96	98	100	102	105	107	109	112	114
41	45	48	50	53	55	57	60	62	65	67	70	72	74	77	79	81	84	86	89	91	93	96	98	100	103	105	108	110	112	115	117	120
42	46	50	53	56	58	60	63	65	68	70	73	75	78	80	83	85	88	90	93	95	98	100	103	105	108	110	113	115	118	120	123	126
43	50	53	55	58	60	63	66	68	71	74	76	79	82	84	87	89	92	95	97	100	103	105	108	110	113	115	118	121	124	126	129	132
44	52	55	58	61	63	66	69	72	74	77	80	83	85	88	91	94	96	99	102	105	107	110	113	116	121	124	127	129	132	130	138	
45	55	58	60	63	66	69	72	75	78	81	84	86	89	92	96	98	101	104	107	109	112	115	118	121	124	127	130	133	135	138	141	144
46	57	60	63	66	69	72	75	78	81	84	87	90	93	96	99	102	105	108	111	114	117	120	123	126	129	132	135	138	141	144	147	150
47	60	63	66	69	72	76	79	82	85	88	91	94	97	101	104	107	110	113	116	119	123	126	129	132	135	138	141	145	148	151	154	157
48	62	66	69	72	75	79	82	85	88	92	95	98	102	105	108	111	115	118	121	125	128	131	134	138	141	144	147	151	154	157	161	164
49	65	69	72	75	79	82	85	89	92	96	99	102	106	109	113	116	120	123	126	130	133	137	140	143	147	150	154	157	161	164	167	171
50	58	71	75	78	82	85	89	92	96	100	103	107	110	114	117	121	124	128	132	135	139	142	146	149	153	156	160	164	167	171	174	178
51	70	74	78	81	85	89	92	96	100	104	107	111	115	118	122	126	129	133	137	141	144	148	152	155	159	163	166	170	174	178	181	185
52	73	77	81	85	88	92	96	100	104	108	112	115	119	123	127	131	135	138	142	146	150	154	158	162	165	169	173	177	181	185	188	192
53	76	80	84	88	92	96	100	104	108	112	116	120	124	128	132	136	140	144	148	152	156	160	164	168	172	176	180	184	188	192	196	200
54	79	83	87	91	95	100	104	108	112	116	120	124	129	133	137	141	145	149	153	158	162	166	170	174	178	182	187	191	195	199	203	207
55	82	86	90	95	99	103	108	112	116	120	125	129	133	138	142	146	151	155	159	164	168	172	176	181	185	189	194	198	202	207	211	215
56	85	89	94	98	103	107	112	116	120	125	129	134	138	143	147	152	156	161	165	170	174	178	183	187	192	196	201	205	210	214	219	223
57	88	92	97	102	106	111	116	120	125	129	134	139	143	148	153	157	162	166	171	176	180	185	189	194	198	203	208	213	217	222	226	231
58	91	96	100	105	110	115	120	124	129	134	139	144	148	153	158	163	167	172	177	182	187	191	196	201	206	211	215	220	225	230	234	239
59	94	99	104	109	114	119	124	128	133	138	144	149	154	158	163	168	173	178	183	188	193	198	203	208	213	218	223	228	233	238	243	248
60	97	102	108	113	118	123	128	133	138	143	149	154	159	164	169	174	179	184	189	195	200	205	210	215	220	225	230	236	241	246	251	256

A child greater than 60 inches tall can be plotted utilizing an adult BMI Table.

Pennsylvania Dietetic Association
An Affiliate of the American Dietetic Association
PO Box 60870 ~ Harrisburg, PA 17106-0870~ (717) 236-1220
www.eatrightpa.org

Summary

In order for your children to have the best results, live a healthy, long life and be physically and mentally fit, they need to have a good beginning.

Before pregnancy, try to maintain a normal weight and avoid cigarettes, alcohol and drugs. Otherwise, the chemicals from these habits could adversely affect your child.

Remember food is a drug. If you are overweight, you increase your child's chances of being obese and developing diabetes, vascular disease and cancer at a young age. They will also be prone to more infections and allergies. Cigarettes, alcohol and drugs will affect their brain and the rest of their organs.

If your BMI is greater than 25, you can still turn things around during pregnancy by following a high nutrient diet and weighing yourself daily. You should also exercise regularly.

Once the child is born, the best gift you can give your child is to breast-feed for as long as possible, up to two years. With a lot of women in the workforce today, it can be difficult. Six to nine months of breast-feeding may be all that's possible, but try to do the best that you can. The child is likely to be much healthier if they are breast-fed. Essentially, you will be giving your child a head start.

With the knowledge you have gained, you can start your child on a healthy eating track at two years of age. Be tough and set a good example. Your child's taste buds will not like fatty foods if they never eat them.

Take walks with your children and allow them to experience nature. Teach them about sports, and help them pick a lifetime sport. At age 73, I practice yoga and play tennis three times each week. I started at a very young age and my general health is excellent.

Use the BMI charts, starting at age two. Weigh and measure your child at least once a month, or every two weeks if they have a problem.

Do the same for yourself. That way you can take good care of your own health and set an example for your children.

Be especially vigilant about what your children are eating. Decide on the general program you will follow: vegetarian, vegan, flexitarian or nutritarian. You have enough knowledge now to do it. If you follow this program 80 to 90% of the time, you will live a very healthy life.

If there are genetic factors, such as parents dying at a young age from diabetes or vascular disease, you will need to be very strict about what you eat and what you are teaching your children.

Remember, the secret of the Non Diet is a way of eating, not a diet. Eat until you are full, not stuffed. You don't have to be perfect, just eat that way the majority of the time.

Underline important points in this book and reread them on a monthly basis, until it is well established in your mind. These are general principles that are not difficult to follow. You may need to seek social support. Remember the Western diet is the worst diet in the world. Don't eat like your friends, unless they're extremely lucky, many of them will get the usual Western illnesses: heart disease, strokes, cancer, diabetes, metabolic syndrome and infectious diseases.

Yesterday, a lady came up to me and said she lost 100 pounds following the secrets of the Non Diet. Please feel free to contact me with your results. I read and collect them.

Good luck!

www.kachmanmindbody.com
(260) 420-YOGA

CDC Growth Charts: United States

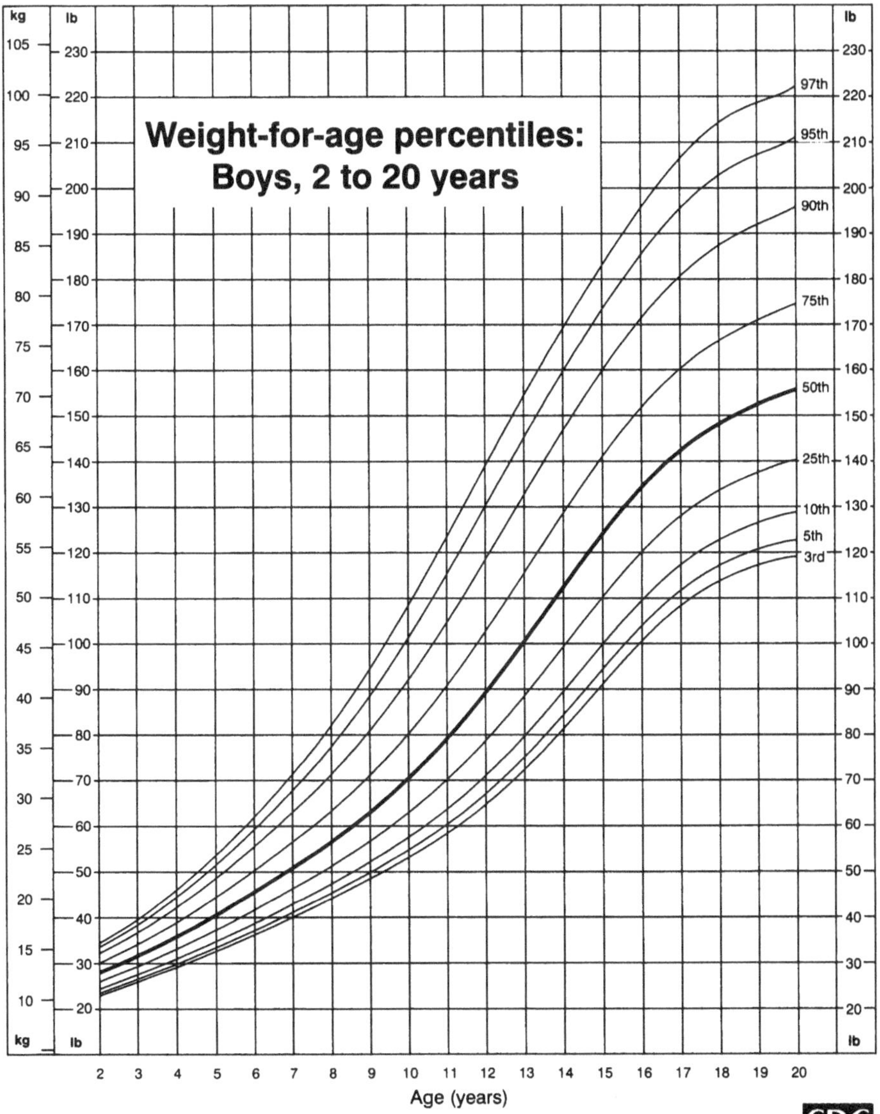

**Weight-for-age percentiles:
Boys, 2 to 20 years**

Age (years)

Published May 30, 2000.
SOURCE: Developed by the National Center for Health Statistics in collaboration with
the National Center for Chronic Disease Prevention and Health Promotion (2000).

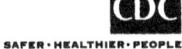

CDC Growth Charts: United States

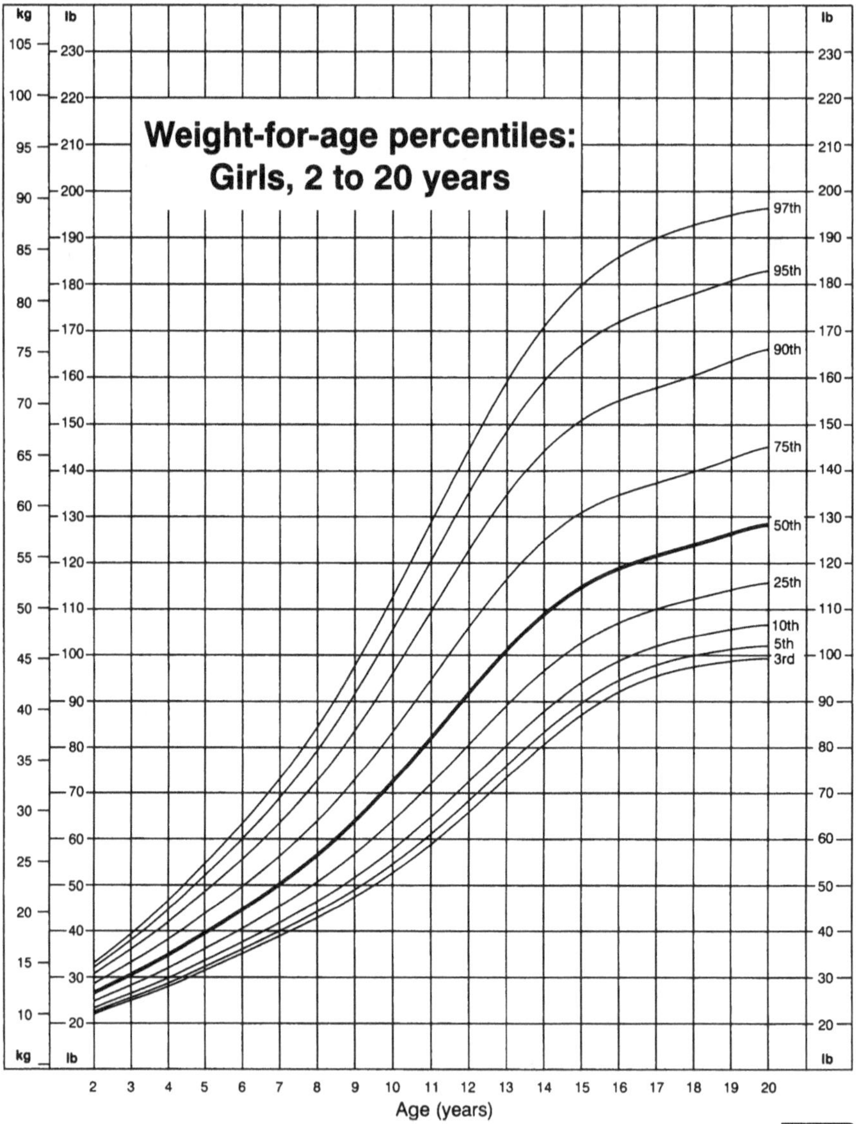

Weight-for-age percentiles: Girls, 2 to 20 years

97th
95th
90th
75th
50th
25th
10th
5th
3rd

Age (years)

Published May 30, 2000.
SOURCE: Developed by the National Center for Health Statistics in collaboration with
the National Center for Chronic Disease Prevention and Health Promotion (2000).

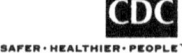

CDC
SAFER · HEALTHIER · PEOPLE™

Adult Body Fat and BMI Numbers For Men and Women

BMI Ratios

Men	Women	Risk Factor
BMI Less Than 20.1	BMI Less than 19.1	Underweight, Lower BMI=greater risk
20.1 to 26.4	19.1 to 25.8	Nomal, very low risk
26.4 to 27.8	25.8 to 27.3	Marginally overweight, some risk
27.8 to 31.1	27.3 to 32.2	Overweight, moderate risk
31.1 to 45.4	32.3 to 44.8	Severe overweight, high risk
Greater than 45.4	Greater than 44.8	Morbid obesity, very high risk

Body Fat Percentage for Men

Ideal Body Fat Percentage for Men				
Age	Excellent	Good	Fair	Risky
20-24	10.8	14.9	19	23.3
25-29	12.8	16.5	20.3	24.3
30-34	14.5	18	21.5	25.2
35-39	16.1	19.3	22.6	26.1
40-44	17.5	20.5	23.6	26.9
45-49	18.6	21.5	24.5	27.6
50-54	19.5	22.3	25.2	28.3
55-59	20	22.9	25.9	28.9
60+	20.3	23.4	26.4	29.5

Body Fat Percentage for Women

Ideal Body Fat Percentage for Women				
Age	Excellent	Good	Fair	Risky
20-24	18.9	22	25	29.6
25-29	18.9	22.1	25.4	29.8
30-34	19.7	22.7	26.4	30.5
35-39	21	24	27.7	31.5
40-44	22.6	25.6	29.3	32.8
45-49	24.3	27.3	30.9	34.1
50-54	25.8	28.9	32.3	35.5
55-59	27	30.2	33.5	36.7
60+	27.6	30.9	34.2	37.7

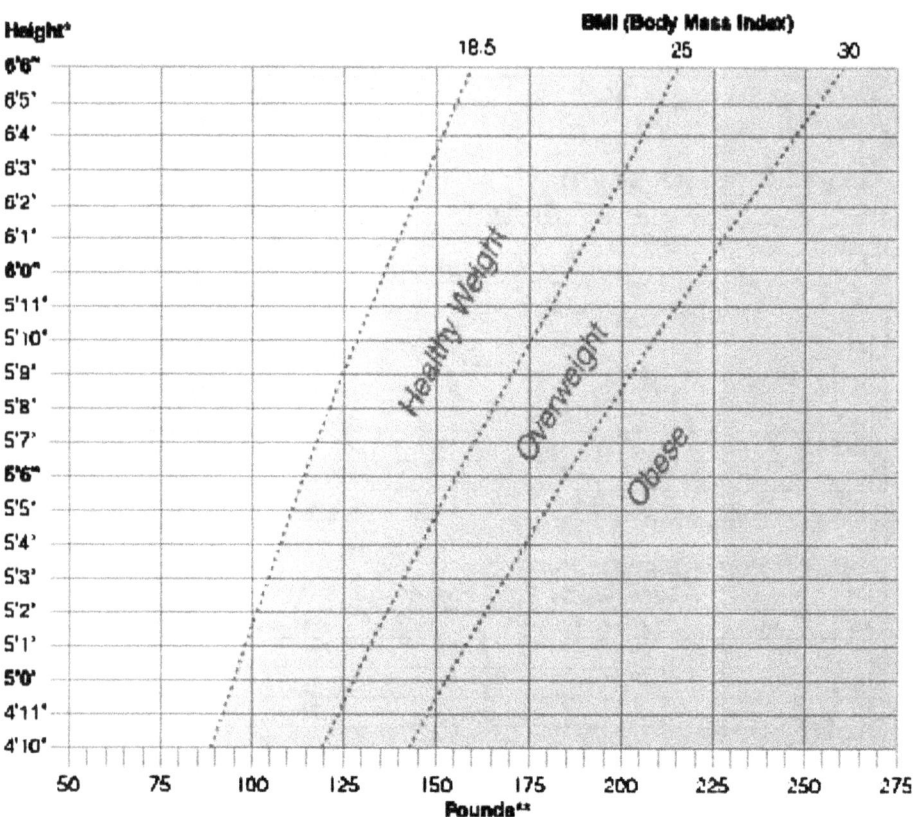

KIDS PANCAKE FUN

Kids love to make this recipe with mom and dad let them have fun mixing all these great healthy breakfast items and throw in a few surprises! It is also fun to use pancake molds to create great pancake shapes to eat.

INGREDIENTS:
½ cup Kashi GOLEAN High Fiber Protein Cereal
¼ cup oat bran
1 Tbsp whole oats
1 Tbsp your child's favorite cereal
¼ cup your child's favorite berries (blueberries are great!)
2 egg whites
1 Tbsp all natural sugar-free applesauce
1 Tbsp Splenda
¼ cup milk
Pinch of salt
½ tsp cinnamon (optional)

PREPARATION: Mix all ingredients well with fork until completely mixed. Optional: ad water for desired consistency. Cook in pan lightly sprayed with Parkay spray butter.

NUTRITIONAL INFO: Makes 4 pancakes: 250 calories, 1 g fat, 37 carbs, 24 g protein, 12g fiber

ORGANIC BEAN BURRITOS

INGREDIENTS:
1 medium Aztecan burrito shell
¼ cup fat-free organic refried beans.
¼ cup fat-free shredded cheddar cheese
2 Tbsp each salsa & fat-free sour cream

PREPARATION: Spread all ingredients on half tortilla. Fold in half and cook in a dry pan 1 minute on both sides or until golden. Enjoy with fat-free sour cream and additional salsa on the side.

NUTRITIONAL INFO: Serves 1: 215 cal, 2.5g fat, 32g carb, 3g fiber, 16g protein

OATMEAL COOKIES

INGREDIENTS:
2 cups oatmeal or oat bran
2 cups Splenda
4 egg whites
1 cup low fat ricotta cheese
1 Tbsp cinnamon
¼ tsp salt
1/8 tsp baking powder – optional (for rising)
½ cup chocolate chips – optional

PREPARATION: Preheat oven to 425 ° F. Mix Splenda, oatmeal, cinnamon, salt, baking powder and chips; set aside. Mix egg whites, ricotta cheese and then combine all ingredients. Spoon onto un-greased baking sheet and bake for 8-10 minutes or until golden brown.

NUTRITIONAL INFO: Makes 24 cookies, amount per cookie: 50 cal, 11g carb, 1g fiber, 2g protein

QUICK CHEESE PIZZA

INGREDIENTS:
1 Azteca Flour Tortilla (medium size)
½ cup Maria Thomas Marinara
Sprinkle of fat-free Parmesan cheese
¼ cup fat-free shredded mozzarella cheese

PREPARATION: Preheat oven to 400°F. Place tortillas on cookie sheet or pizza tray and spread marinara on tortilla; sprinkle each with cheese. Bake for 6-8 minutes until crust crispy and cheese is melted. Keep an eye on them—they cook fast! Cool for 5 minutes and serve.

NUTRITIONAL INFO: Serves 1: 180 calories, 2.5 g. fat, 24 g. carbs, 13 g. protein

QUICK HEALTHY FRENCH FRIES

INGREDIENTS:
1 large baking potato, sweet potato or red potato
Salt, Old Bay & garlic salt to taste
Parkay Spray Butter

PREPARATION: Preheat oven to 425° F. Slice potato into French fries pieces. Coat cookie sheet with spray butter and spread potatoes on cookie sheet, 1 layer. Sprinkle with salt, Old Bay seasoning, and garlic salt; bake for 10-15 minutes or until golden brown.

NUTRITIONAL INFO: 4 servings, per serving: 32 calories, 1 g. fiber, 8 g. carbs

END NOTES

[1] Walter Willett, M.D., Fredrick John Stare Professor of Epidemiology and Nutrition, Harvard School of Public Health, and professor of medicine, Harvard Medical School, Boston.

[2] National Center for Health Statistics, *National Vital Statistics Reports*; 53: 17; 2005.

[3] "Role of inflammation—Growing proof inflammation is a major risk factor for heart disease," Cleveland Clinic Heart & Vascular Institute Web site, August, 2002.

[4] P.M. Ridker, et al., "Comparison of C-Reactive Protein and Low-Density Lipoprotein Cholesterol Levels in the Prediction of First Cardiovascular Events," *New England Journal of Medicine*, 347:1557; 2002.

[5] Mora, S., et al., "Physical Activity and Reduced Risk of Cardiovascular Events: Potential Mediating Mechanisms," *Circulation*; 116: 2110 – 2118; 2007.

[6] Campbell, T. Colin, *The China Study: The Most Comprehensive Study of Nutrition Ever Conducted and the Startling Implications for Diet, Weight Loss and Long-term Health*, Benbella Books, 2006.

[7] Nissen, Steven E., M.D., et al., *The New England Journal of Medicine*, 352:29; 2005.

[8] Ornish, D., et al., "Can lifestyle changes reverse coronary heart disease? The Lifestyle Heart Trial," *Lancet*; Jul 21; 336 (8708):129-33; 1990.

[9] Esselstyn, Caldwell B., Jr., *Prevent and Reverse Heart Disease*, Avery, 2007.

[10] Centers for Disease Control and Prevention, National Health Center for Statistics, "Obesity Still a Major Problem," April 14, 2006.

[11] Convit, A., "Hypothalamic-Pituitary-Adrenal Axis Dysregulation and Memory Impairments in Type 2 diabetes," *The Journal of Clinical Endocrinology & Metabolism*; Vol. 92, No. 7 2439-2445; 2007.

[12] Zhang, C., et al., "Abdominal Obesity and the Risk of All-Cause, Cardiovascular, and Cancer Mortality: Sixteen Years of Follow-Up in US Women," *Circulation*, Apr 2008; 117: 1658 - 1667.

[13] Pollan, M., "Unhappy Meals," *The New York Times Magazine*, January 28, 2007.

[14] Ibid, Campbell, C.

[15] World Health Organization, Joint WHO/FAO Expert Consultation "Diet, Nutrition and the Prevention of Chronic Diseases," WHO Technical Report Series 916; 2003.

[16] Chandalia M. et al., "Beneficial effects of high dietary fiber intake in patients with type 2 diabetes mellitus," *New England Journal of Medicine*; 342:1392-1398; 2000.

[17] Slyper, A., "Influence of glycemic load on HDL cholesterol in youth," *American Journal of Clinical Nutrition*; 81: 2, 376-379; 2005.

[18] Jacobs, D., *American Journal of Clinical Nutrition*; 68: 248, 1998.

[19] Pollan, Michael, *In Defense of Food*, Penguin Press, 2008.

[20] Aviram M, Rosenblat M, Gaitini D, et al, "Pomegranate juice consumption for 3 years by patients with carotid artery stenosis reduces common carotid intima-media thickness, blood pressure and LDL oxidation," *Clin Nutr* 23 (3): 423–33; June, 2004.

[21] Studer, M., "Effect of Different Antilipidemic Agents and Diets on Mortality: A Systematic Review," *The Archives of Internal Medicine*; 165:725 – 730; 2005.

[22] AP, Simopoulos, "Omega-3 fatty acids in health and disease and in growth and development," *Am J Clin Nutr*; 54:438-63; 1991.

[23] Katan MB, et al., "Trans fatty acids and their effects on lipoproteins in humans," *Annual Review of Nutrition*; 15:473-93; 1995.

[24] Rafferty, J., "Trans Fat 'Ban Wagon,'" *Harvard Public Health Review*, http://www.hsph.harvard.edu/review/spring07/spr07transfat.html; 2007.

[25] Ascherio A, Stampfer MJ, Willett WC, "Trans fatty acids and coronary heart disease," Harvard School of Public Health, http://www.hsph.harvard.edu/; 2006.

[26] Wilson, M., "Carbohydrates, Proteins, and Fats," *Merck Manual of Medical Information*, http://www.merck.com/mmhe/print/sec12/ch152/ch152b.html; 2008.

[27] Pischon, T., *The New England Journal of Medicine*; 359:2105-2120; 2008.

[28] Ibid, Willett, W.

[29] U.S. Department of Agriculture, *Economic Research Service Briefing*, May 25, 2007.

[30] Fleming, R., "The effect of high-protein diets on coronary blood flow," *Angiography*; 51 (10):817-26; 2000.

[31] Ibid, Campbell.

[32] Ob cit, Campbell.

[33] Kuo, P., "Angina pectoris induced by fat ingestion in patients with coronary artery disease," *Journal of the American Medical Association*; 1008-1013; July 23, 1955.

[34] Esselstyn, C., "Resolving the Coronary Artery Disease Epidemic through Plant-Based Nutrition," *Preventative Cardiology*; 4: 171-177; 2001.

[35] Tsai AG, Wadden, et al., "Systematic review: an evaluation of major commercial weight loss programs in the United States," *Annals of Internal Medicine*; 142 (1):56-66; 2005.

[36] Dansinger ML et al., "Comparison of the Atkins, Ornish, Weight Watchers and Zone diets for weight loss and heart disease risk reduction: a randomized trial,: *JAMA* ;293: 43–53; 2005.

[37] Brownell, K., "Fighting Obesity and the Food Lobby," *The Washington Post*, June 9, 2002; Page B07.

[38] CDC, National Center for Health Statistics, National Health and Nutrition Examination Survey, *Journal of the American Medical Association*, 2002; 288:1723-7; 2002.

[39] Olshansky, J., "A Potential Decline in Life Expectancy in the United States in the 21st Century," *New England Journal of Medicine*; 352:1138-1145; 2005.

[40] Deakin University; "Study Shows Fruit Juice/Drink Link to Children's Weight Gain," *Science Daily*, 29 March 2007.

[41] Libby, P., "Atherosclerosis: the New View," *Scientific Am.*; 286 (5):46-55; May; 2002.

[42] Libby, P., "The molecular mechanisms of the thrombotic complications of atherosclerosis," *Journal of Internal Medicine*; 263(5):517-27; May 2008.

[43] P.M. Ridker, et al., "C-reactive protein and other markers of inflammation in the prediction of cardiovascular disease in women," *New England Journal of Medicine*, 342(12):836-43, 2000.

[44] Robinson, Joshua, "After Completing Marathon, a Runner Dies in His Home," *The New York Times*, November 7, 2007.

[45] Kandel, E., *In Search of Memory: The Emergence of a New Science of Mind*, W.W. Norton, 2007.

[46] Garrison, Julia Fox, *Don't Leave Me This Way*, Harper Collins, 2007.

[47] Cheng, M., "Studies Tout Treating Mini-Strokes Fast," *Brain in the News*, November 2007.

[48] Ibid, Cheng.

[50] Women and cardiovascular diseases statistics, American Heart Association, 2004.

[51] Kolata, G., "Reversing Trend, Big Drop Is Seen in Breast Cancer," *The New York Times*, December 15, 2006.

[52] Miller, A.P, et al., "Secondary Prevention of Coronary Heart Disease in Women: A Call to Action," *Annals of Internal Medicine*; 138 2 81-160; 2001.

[53] Cook, N., et al., "Physical Activity and Reduced Risk of Cardiovascular Events: Potential Mediating Mechanisms," *Circulation: Journal of the American Heart Association*; 116: 2110 – 2118; 2007.

[54] P. Barberger-Gateau, et al., "Dietary patterns and risk of dementia," *Neurology*, 69:1921-1930; 2007.

[55] Morris, Martha C.; Sacks, Frank; Rosner, Bernard, Does fish oil lower blood pressure? A meta-analysis of controlled trials," *Circulation*; 88 (2): 523–533; 1993.

[56] Sanders, T., et al., "Influence of n–6 versus n–3 polyunsaturated fatty acids in diets low in saturated fatty acids on plasma lipoproteins and hemostatic factors," *Arteriosclerosis, Thrombosis, and Vascular Biology*; 17 (12): 3449–3460; 1997.

[57] National Health and Nutrition Examination Survey (NHANES), 1999-2004, National Center for Health Statistics and the NHLBI.

[58] Esselstyn, C., *Prevent and Reverse Heart Disease*, Penguin Group, 2007.

[59] Whitaker, Julian, *Reversing Heart Disease*, Warner Books, 2002.

[60] Levy, R., "Report on the Lipid Research Clinic Trials," *European Heart Journal*, E: 45-53; August 1987.

[61] Flegal, K., et al., "Cause-specific excess deaths associated with underweight, overweight, and obesity," *Journal of American Medical Association*; 298: 2028-2037; 2007.

[62] *American College of Radiology* press release, "Zoos Stretched to Limit as Providers Seek Supersized Scanners for Morbidly Obese Patients," 2008.

[63] Frazao, E. et al., "America's eating habits: changes and consequences," USDA/ERS Agri. Info. Bull. 750; 1999.

[64] Cutler, D., et al., "Why Have Americans Become More Obese?" *The Economics of Obesity*; Economic Research Service/USDA.

[65] Wilson, P. et al., *Archives of Internal Medicine*; 162: 1867-1872; 2002.

[66] Ezzati, M., et al., "Causes of cancer in the world: comparative risk assessment of nine behavioral and environmental risk factors," *The Lancet*; 366:1784–1793; 2005.

[67] Lutsey, P., "Dietary Intake and the Development of the Metabolic Syndrome," *Circulation*; 117:754-761; 2008.

[68] "Dietary Intake and the Development of the Metabolic Syndrome," *Circulation*; 117:754-761; 2008.

[69] "Pre-diabetes," Mayo Clinic.com, Jan. 5, 2008.

[70] Kaufman, F., *Diabesity*, Bantam Books, 2005.

[71] National Diabetes Statistics; National Institutes for Health; 2005.

[72] Ibid, Kaufman, F.

[73] Brody, Jane E., "'Diabesity,' a Crisis in an Expanding Country," *The New York Times*, March 29, 2005.

[74] Jensen, M., "Intakes of whole grains, bran, and germ and the risk of coronary heart disease in men," *American Journal of Clinical Nutrition*; 80: 6, 1492-1499; 2004.

[75] Sachiko, T., et al., Statement of the AHA Nutrition Committee; *Circulation*; 104:1869; 2001.

[76] "Reduction of Type 2 Diabetes with Lifestyle Interventions," *New England Journal of Medicine*; 346: 393-403; 2002.

[77] "Long-term Effects of Renin-Angiotensin System–Blocking Therapy and a Low Blood Pressure Goal on Progression of Hypertensive Chronic Kidney Disease in African-Americans," *Arch Intern Med.*; 168(8):832-839; 2008.

[78] 10 ways to control high blood pressure without medication, MayoClinic.com, May 21, 2008.

[79] Flack, J., "Epidemiology of Hypertension and Cardiovascular Disease in African-Americans," *The Journal of Clinical Hypertension*; Volume 5 Issue 1 Page 5-11; 2003.

[80] Benjamin EJ, et al., "Evidence-Based Guidelines for Cardiovascular Disease Prevention in Women: 2007 Update," *Circulation*; 2007.

[81] Fuhrman, Joel, *Eat to Live*, Little, Brown, & Co., 2003.

[82] High Blood Pressure Statistics, American Heart Association.org, 2008.

[83] Guimont, C., et al., "Chronic job strain may raise blood pressure," *American Journal of Public Health*, August 2006.

[84] Ruiz, J., et al., "Association between muscular strength and mortality in men: prospective cohort study," *British Medical Journal*; 337:a439;2008.

[85] Didion, J., *The Year of Magical Thinking*, Knopf, 2005.

[86] Bajaj, V. "An Enron Chapter Closes: An Obituary; Kenneth L. Lay, 64, Enron Founder and Symbol of Corporate Excess," *The New York Times*, July 5, 2006.

[87] Shedd, O., et al., "The World Trade Center attack: Increased frequency of defibrillator shocks for ventricular arrhythmias in patients living remotely from New York City," *Journal of the American College of Cardiology*; vol. 44: 6, pp. 1265-1267; 2004.

[88] Guarneri, M., *The Heart Speaks*, Touchstone, 2006.

[89] Lavelle, P. "Anger trigger to heart disease found?" *ABC Science Online*, 2003.

[90] World Health Organization, "The World Health Report 2001: Mental Health: New Understanding, New Hope."

[91] Nielsen, KM, "Danish singles have a twofold risk of acute coronary syndrome," *Journal of Epidemiology and Community Health*; 60:721-728; 2006.

[92] Hughes, J., *American Heart Journal*, May 2006.

[93] Bagga D, et al., "Effects of a very low fat, high fiber diet on serum hormones and menstrual function," *Cancer*; 76:2491-6; 1995.

[94] Gureje, O., et al., "Persistent Pain and Well-being: A World Health Organization Study in Primary Care," *Journal of American Medical Association*, 280(2): 147-51, 1998.

[95] Ornish, D., "Love Is Real Medicine," *Newsweek*, October 3, 2005.

[96] Goleman, D., *Social Intelligence: The New Science of Human Relationships*, Bantam, 2006.

[97] Blakeslee, S., "Cells that Read Minds," *The New York Times*, January 10, 2006.

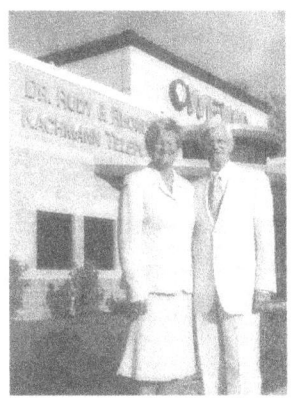

Rudy Kachmann, M.D., is the cofounder of the Kachmann Mind Body Institute in Fort Wayne, Indiana, and has been in practice for over 40 years. Dr. Kachmann received his Neurosurgery training from Georgetown University. He received his M.D. and a B.S. in Chemistry from Indiana University.

His major interests are wellness and holistic healing. He has been on PBS and his lectures have been broadcast on PBS. He is a regular lecturer on subjects of the mind body including diet, stress, cancer, back pain and Asian healing. He lectures to corporations and includes stress and finances lectures. He is regularly featured in local media, including radio shows, doing a regular monthly television broadcast called "Docs on Call," newspapers, magazines and medical journals. He is the author of *Twenty Prescriptions for Living the Good Life*, *Welcome to Your Mind Body*, DVDs on mind body, back pain, a DVD lecture series and producer of *Oh My Aching Back*.

Dr. Kachmann is on the Board of Directors of Day Break Children's Shelter and the Board of Trustees of Lutheran Hospital. He is the founder of the Kachmann Behavioral Foundation that funds community-based educational initiatives, and is a member of the Tennis Hall of Fame. He has received several awards, including the Martin Luther King award for his support of community outreach. Dr. Kachmann is a long-time resident of Fort Wayne where he lives with his wife, Yorkshire terrier and two Tonkinese cats.

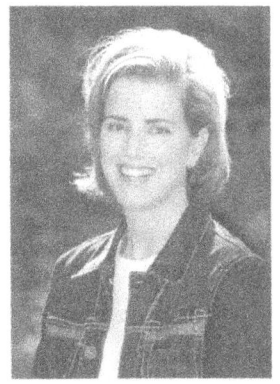

Kim Kachmann-Geltz received a B.A. in humanities from Indiana University and a M.A. in American Studies from Columbia University. Her writing career began as a legislative correspondent on Capitol Hill. Her knowledge of health care and medicine grew as the director of SpeakOutUSA, a non-profit that developed educational videos and produced health care reform hearings for bipartisan members of the U.S. Congress.

She joined America Online, Inc. as writer and editor of the "Welcome Screen" before becoming director of AOL International Content & Programming. There she developed the company's first manual on editorial content standards, practices and taught the "best practices" to AOL's joint ventures in 11 different countries around the world.

She lives on Hilton Head Island with her husband, three young children, Yorkshire terrier, rabbit and two Tonkinese cats.

The Kachmann Mind Body Institute is the leader in research, education, and clinical practice of mind body medicine. We teach various complementary mind body therapies as the ultimate integrative and holistic approach to healing. We recognize the connection between human experience, self awareness and one's health. Not only are we interested in helping build a healthy immune system, but we are interested in helping build a healthy mind. We help individuals understand how the mind and body are interconnected and how they function as a whole.

The Kachmann Mind Body Institute is dedicated to helping individuals create and maintain lifelong health through various mind body programs including:

- Group Yoga & Fitness Classes & Workshops
- Weight Management
- Personal Fitness Training
- Holistic Pain Management
- Yoga Therapy
- Massage Therapy
- Corporate Wellness
- Dr. Rudy Kachmann Lecture Series
- Physician Consultation

Lutheran Hospital Campus
7900 West Jefferson Blvd.
Suite 108 MOB1
Fort Wayne, IN 46804

Downtown Fort Wayne
1301 Layette St.
Suite 205
Fort Wayne, IN 46802

For more information please contact us at 260-420-YOGA (9642) or visit www.KachmannMindBody.com

Other Books and Media from Dr. Kachmann

You may purchase these products at www.kachmannmindbody.com

BOOKS

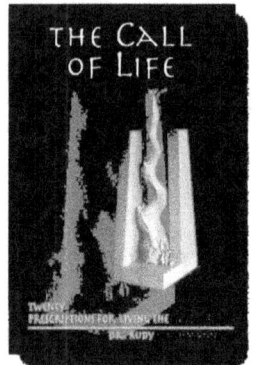 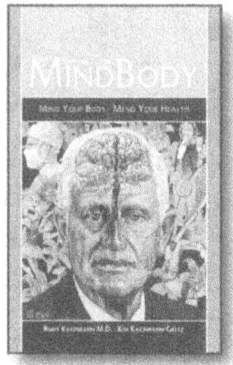 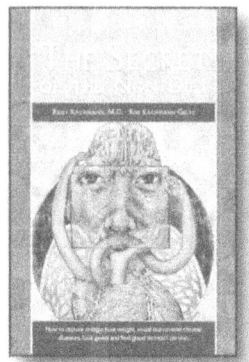

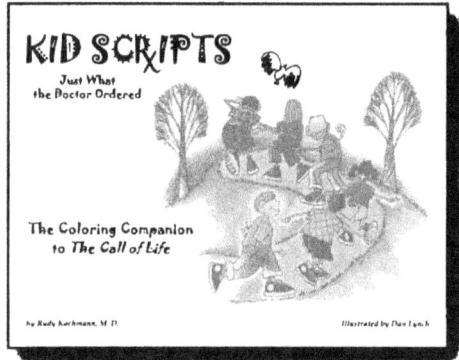

DVDS

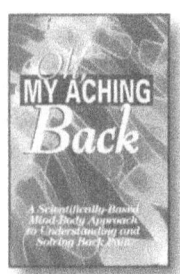 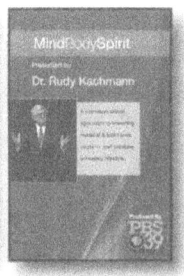 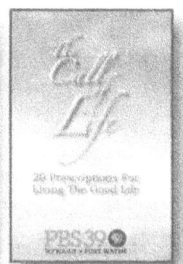 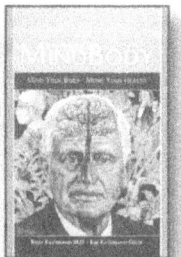 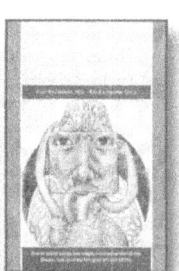

COMING SOON

Nocebo the Evil Twin

The Secret of the Non Diet for Children (DVD)
The Secret of Living Healthier Longer (DVD)
The Mind and Stress (DVD)
Placebo Nocebo (DVD)